TREATING
LANGUAGE DISORDERS

Dedicated to the memory of Wendell Johnson—
humanist, scientist, clinician,
statesman for the profession

FOR CLINICIANS BY CLINICIANS
Harris Winitz, Series Editor

This book, **Treating Language Disorders**, inaugurates the **FOR CLINICIANS
BY CLINICIANS** series of texts on the diagnosis and clinical management of
speech, language, and voice disorders. Each text provides a contemporary
perspective of one major disorder or clinical area, and is designed for use in
clinical methodology courses and continuing education programs. Authors
have been selected who represent a broad spectrum of clinical interests and
theoretical positions, but who hold the common belief that their viewpoints,
experiences, and successes should be shared in order to provide a forum **FOR
CLINICIANS BY CLINICIANS.**

TREATING LANGUAGE DISORDERS

FOR CLINICIANS BY CLINICIANS

Edited by
Harris Winitz, Ph.D.
Professor of Communication Studies and Psychology
University of Missouri Kansas City

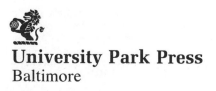

University Park Press
Baltimore

UNIVERSITY PARK PRESS
International Publishers in Medicine and Human Services
300 North Charles Street
Baltimore, Maryland 21201

Copyright © 1983 by University Park Press

Typeset by Maryland Composition Company
Manufactured in the United States of America by
The Maple Press Company

Library of Congress Cataloging in Publication Data
Main entry under title:

Treating language disorders.

Includes bibliographies and index.
1. Language disorders—Treatment. I. Winitz, Harris,
1933–   . [DNLM: 1. Language disorders—Therapy.
WL 340 T784]
RC423.T73   1983   616.85'506   82-23682
ISBN 0-8391-1813-9

Contents

Contributors vii

Preface ix

CHAPTER 1
Are We Training Young Language Delayed Children for
    Future Academic Failure? 1
    Karen F. Steckol

CHAPTER 2
Data Based Language Programs: A Closer Look 11
    Kyla Becker Marion

CHAPTER 3
Use and Abuse of the Developmental Approach 25
    Harris Winitz

CHAPTER 4
Facilitating Comprehension, Recall, and Production
    of Language 43
    Elaine Z. Lasky

CHAPTER 5
Curriculum Concepts for Language Treatment
    of Children 57
    Lawrence J. Turton

CHAPTER 6
Interactive Model for the Assessment and Treatment of
    the Young Child 79
    LuVern H. Kunze, Sarah K. Lockhart, Sharon M.
    Didow, and Mary Caterson

CHAPTER 7
Creating Communicative Context 97
    Catherine M. Constable

CHAPTER **8**
Facilitating Language in Emotionally Handicapped
Children 121
  Amy Belkin

CHAPTER **9**
Language and the Atmosphere of Delight.......................... 143
  R. McCrae Cochrane

CHAPTER **10**
Communication Styles of Fluent Aphasic Clients 163
  Robert C. Marshall

CHAPTER **11**
Minor Hemisphere Mediation in Aphasia Treatment............... 181
  Jennifer Horner and Karen Hardin Fedor

CHAPTER **12**
Vocabulary Selection in Augmentative Communication:
  Where Do We Begin? 205
  Andrea F. Blau

CHAPTER **13**
Microcomputers: A Clinical Aid 235
  Mary S. Wilson and Bernard J. Fox

Index 249

Contributors

Amy Belkin, Ed.D.
Speech-Language Pathologist
Reece School
180 East 93rd Street
New York, New York 10028

Andrea F. Blau, M.S., M.Phil.
Speech and Hearing Sciences
Graduate School and University
    Center
City University of New York
33 West 42nd Street
New York, New York 10036

Mary Caterson, M.S.
Speech Pathologist
Pediatric Rehabilitation
John F. Kennedy Medical Center
Edison, New Jersey 08818

R. McCrae Cochrane, Ph.D.
Director, Communication Disorders
Casa Colina Rehabilitation Hospital
255 East Bonita Avenue
Pomona, California 91767

Catherine M. Constable, M.Ed.
Instructor/Preschool Coordinator
Department of Communication
    Disorders
Bloomsburg State College
Bloomsburg, Pennsylvania 17815

Sharon M. Didow, M.S.
Clinical Speech/Language
    Pathologist
Duke University Medical Center
Center for Speech and Hearing
    Disorders
P.O. Box 3887
Durham, North Carolina 27710

Karen Hardin Fedor, M.S.
Clinical Speech/Language
    Pathologist
Audiology-Speech Pathology Service
Veterans Administration Medical
    Center
Durham, North Carolina 27710

Bernard J. Fox, M.S.
Vice President
Laureate Learning Services Inc.
1 Mill Street
Burlington, Vermont 05405

Jennifer Horner, Ph.D.
Assistant Professor of Speech/
    Language Pathology
Duke University Medical Center
Center for Speech and Hearing
    Disorders
Department of Surgery
P.O. Box 3887
Durham, North Carolina 27710

LuVern H. Kunze, Ph.D.
Professor of Speech/Language
    Pathology
Duke University Medical Center
Center for Speech and Hearing
    Disorders
P.O. Box 3887
Durham, North Carolina 27710

Elaine Z. Lasky, Ph.D.
Professor of Speech and Hearing
Department of Speech and Hearing
Cleveland State University
Cleveland, Ohio 44115

Sarah K. Lockhart, M.S.
Clinical Speech/Language
    Pathologist
Duke University Medical Center
Center for Speech and Hearing
    Disorders
P.O. Box 3887
Durham, North Carolina 27710

Kyla Becker Marion, M.A.
Speech Services Unit of the
  Division of Special Education
Board of Education
New York City
100 Livingston Street
Brooklyn, New York 11201

Robert C. Marshall, Ph.D.
Chief, Audiology and Speech
  Pathology Service
Veterans Administration Center
3710 S.W. U.S. Veterans Hospital
  Road;
Clinical Assistant Professor,
  Neurology
Oregon Health Sciences University
Portland, Oregon 97201

Karen F. Steckol, Ph.D.
Assistant Professor of Surgery
Division of Communicative
  Disorders
Myers Hall
University of Kentucky
Louisville, Kentucky 40292

Lawrence J. Turton, Ph.D.
Associate Professor of Speech
  Pathology
Room 216, Davis Hall
Indiana University of Pennsylvania
Indiana, Pennsylvania 15705

Mary S. Wilson, Ph.D.
Professor
Communication Science and
  Disorders
Allen House
University of Vermont
Burlington, Vermont 05405

Harris Winitz, Ph.D.
Professor of Communication Studies
  and Psychology
University of Missouri-Kansas City
5216 Rockhill Road
Kansas City, Missouri 64110

Preface

Shortly before the manuscript for this volume was submitted for publication I had the good fortune to talk with my friend and colleague, Josef Rohrer, director of language instruction for the Federal Language Bureau of West Germany. In the course of our discussion, he used the term *serious,* after Searle (1967), to describe certain teaching practices at his institution. When he defined this term, I realized that it describes well one of three major dimensions of contemporary models of language instruction and language training.

In recent years, communication has resurfaced as a major theoretical consideration in language teaching. A second construct that is recognized as important pertains to the comprehensibility of the language input. Together these two constructs provide a basis for clinical instruction. In brief, it is now acknowledged that language teaching should have a pragmatic focus, and efforts should be made to ensure that the language input is comprehensible.

There is, however, a third dimension in language teaching that is largely independent of these two constructs. The term Josef Rohrer uses is *serious language.* This term describes language that is real, purposeful, and meaningful to the language learner. Practicing a drill or a dialogue, for example, is serious only to language learners who believe that this method of instruction will teach them language. Conversely, a language training routine that is construed by the language learner as artificial denotes nonserious language, even when the clinician regards the language interaction as having a pragmatic basis. Serious language, then, is authentic language for the language learner.

In language training, serious language has been appreciated, but in general, it has not been emphasized. Among those who spoke of it was Joseph Wepman (1976), although he and others did not use this term. Wepman recognized that without the quality of authenticity, the aphasic patient is only a distant observer, not a serious participant. Others have injected the dimension of seriousness into their proposals for training language delayed children. For example, Holland (1975), and later Lahey and Bloom (1977), developed criteria largely based on the dimension of seriousness for the selection of items for teaching a child's initial lexicon, although they also did not use the term.

In foreign language teaching, the term *serious language* describes Curran's (1976) position, which is that language learning should involve ". . . a whole person relationship in which a person's intellect, volition, instincts and soma are seen as all interwoven and engaged together . . ." (p. 15). Father Curran's position is a far cry from the standard "grammar-translation" method of instruction that is endemic to the American high school and university and is regarded among contemporary psycholinguists as a method to study about language rather than a method to acquire language. Wepman (1976) held the same point of view, for he reasoned that language training for aphasic patients should not be "corrective therapy," but instead should be directed to the "embellishment of thought."

But no discussion on the dimension of seriousness in language training can ignore the writings of Wendell Johnson, to whom this book is dedicated. In his classic text *People in Quandaries,* Johnson (1946) repeatedly emphasized that an effective clinical interaction requires a genuinely interested clinician who is able to create a semantic environment that attends to the attitudes, beliefs, customs, standards, and ideals of the individual. Attention must be given to these considerations, he wrote, if we are to understand communication and effectively promote it in the clinical process.

Each of the 18 contributors to this volume on treating language disorders recognizes the importance of serious language in the clinical process. In Chapters 1 and 2, Karen Steckol and Kyla Marion, respectively, challenge traditional procedures of language training and remark that our success rate will continue to be low unless important changes are made in our theoretical models and clinical routines. I suggest in Chapter 3 that these changes, in particular, should involve a restructuring of the way in which the developmental model of language teaching is currently applied.

In Chapter 4, Elaine Lasky gives careful consideration to the complexity of language learning and its interrelation with thought and communication as a clinical process. These considerations are discussed further by Lawrence Turton, who in Chapter 5 presents a comprehensive model of language intervention that includes goals, strategies for instruction, and procedures for evaluation.

The next three chapters provide practical illustrations of communicatively based language programs. LuVern Kunze, Sarah Lockhart, Sharon Didow, and Mary Caterson in Chapter 6, and Catherine Constable in Chapter 7 comprehensively illustrate clinical procedures for teaching communicative functions to language delayed children. In Chapter 8, Amy Belkin presents a special application of these procedures for the emotionally handicapped child with language disorders.

The next three chapters describe language training procedures as they apply to the aphasic patient. R. McCrae Cochrane focuses on strategies for teaching the spontaneity of language in Chapter 9. In Chapter 10, Robert Marshall addresses the difficulty in communication that fluent aphasics have and also identifies treatment procedures. Jennifer Horner and Karin Fedor in Chapter 11 provide detailed consideration of the functional role of the minor hemisphere and appropriate treatment routines.

In Chapter 12, Andrea Blau puts forth criteria for the selection of an initial lexicon for use in augmentative communication. She considers interpersonal and communicative factors, as well as constraints on the use of symbols and their functional utility.

The concluding chapter, by Mary Wilson and Bernard Fox, gives us a futuristic glimpse of the use of computers in language rehabilitation. It is interesting to speculate about their potential application and degree of acceptance by language clinicians.

REFERENCES

Curran, C. A. 1976. Counseling-Learning in Second Languages. Apple River Press, Apple River, IL.

Holland, A. L. 1975. Language therapy for children: Some thoughts on context and content. J. Speech Hear. Disord. 40:514–523.

Johnson, W. 1946. People in Quandaries: The Semantics of Personal Adjustment. Harper and Brothers, New York.

Lahey, M., and Bloom, L. 1977. Planning a first lexicon: Which words to teach first. J. Speech Hear. Disord. 42:340–350.

Searle, J. R. 1967. Speech Acts: An Essay in the Philosophy of Language. Cambridge University Press, New York.

Wepman, J. M. 1976. Aphasia: Language without thought or thought without language. Asha, 18:131–136.

CHAPTER 1

Are We Training Young Language Delayed Children for Future Academic Failure?

Karen F. Steckol

Steckol states that after many years of treatment, language delayed children have difficulty using language in a communicatively appropriate way. The author provides an explanation for their deficiency and puts forward the claim that naturalness should be injected into clinical intervention programs.

1. *Distinguish between the vertical and horizontal approaches of language teaching. Which method do you endorse?*
2. *What are the pitfalls of "packaged language programs" when used with language delayed children? If you use a packaged program, defend your use of it.*
3. *Why does Steckol advocate the use of "naturalness" in the treatment of language? What current approaches does she consider to be natural, and which ones unnatural? How would you apply the concept of naturalness?*
4. *Why does Steckol decide on "play therapy" as a general model for teaching language? Is play therapy a structured or unstructured approach? Is play therapy a stimulus-response model?*

DEPENDING ON ONE'S SCHOOL OF THOUGHT, each person has a particular language intervention technique that seems to be more successful than another. There are many to choose from, and often the choice is a difficult one. When clinicians are asked which intervention model they prefer, discussions almost always center around some form of stimulus-response intervention technique. Although there seem to be an infinite number of derivatives of the stimulus-response format, the ultimate goal in all cases is to increase the child's expressive language to an age appropriate level of functioning. How to arrive at that goal is of major concern.

It would be impossible and impractical to expand on every instructional method that uses the stimulus-response format as a base. This chapter, therefore, describes only two of the widely used stimulus-response techniques and their strengths and weaknesses. The tightest scrutiny is reserved for the question of how these techniques, which have the same goal, prepare the young language delayed child for later academic success or failure. In other words, by using the stimulus-response model, are we training young language delayed children to become language-learning disabled children when they reach school age?

The stimulus-response model takes the form of antecedent event (stimulus)—child's response—consequent event (reinforcement). The antecedent and consequent events are manipulated by the clinician and are intended to shape the child's responses in a positive direction. Stimulus items vary from method to method. Most include pictures, objects, and other symbols. These stimulus items, along with the clinician's verbal directions, stimulus questions, and utterances, provide the antecedent events. The most important aspect of training is the reinforcement that is chosen. Although there are a variety of reinforcement techniques that promote learning (more on this later), generally speaking, most clinicians choose to provide tangible reinforcement (e.g., tokens or food), verbal praise, or some combination of both.

Given the basic training routine mentioned above, let's now focus our attention on some of the more widely used techniques that have the stimulus-response format. The first technique is based on a developmental approach to language remediation. We know that normal speaking children acquire language in a rather systematic fashion. Using the stimulus-response model, we lead language delayed children through the various levels of language development. The goal is to teach mastery of the linguistic structures that are deficient. There are two alternatives within this developmental approach that a clinician can take. One is called the horizontal approach, and the other is denoted the vertical approach.

VERTICAL AND HORIZONTAL DEVELOPMENTAL APPROACHES

In the vertical model a particular linguistic construction type from the child's actual level of functioning is taken to its most advanced state, disregarding other linguistic elements. An example of the vertical approach will help to clarify its usage. Let's take the development of grammatical morphemes to illustrate this point.

Grammatical morphemes are acquired by normal children in a relatively fixed order (Brown, 1973). The *progressive ending -ing* emerges at approximately 2½ years of age, next come *in* and *on,* then *plurals,* then *irregular past tense* (e.g., went), then *possessives,* then the *uncontractible copula* (e.g., Francis *is* happy in which the copula *is* cannot be contracted to form " Francis' happy), then *articles,* then the *regular past tense -ed,* then *regular third person singular, present tense* (e.g., wants), then *irregular third person singular* (e.g., does), then the *uncontractible auxiliary* (e.g., Francis *is* running), then the *contractible copula* (e.g., he *is* happy, for which the contraction is he's happy), and finally, by approximately 4 years of age, the child has mastered the *contractible auxiliary* (e.g., he is running, for which the contraction is he's running). Using the vertical approach, a clinician teaches the *-ing* ending first, then *in, on,* later plurals, and last the contractible auxiliary. One possible developmental training sequence might be as follows:

Level	I	man
Level	II	man sit
Level	III	man sitt*ing*
Level	IV	man sitting chair
Level	V	man sitting *on* chair
Level	VI	*the* man sitting on chair
Level	VII	the man sitting on *the* chair
Level	VIII	the man *is* sitting on the chair

With this intervention format, four grammatical morphemes (*ing, on,* the article *the,* and the contractible auxiliary *is*) are trained in a particular syntactic context. Obviously, not all grammatical morphemes are presented, but each new grammatical morpheme is added, according to the order in which it occurs in the developmental sequence. In addition, the utterances are semantically meaningful throughout, and utterance length is increased by only one morpheme per level. Other vertical developmental sequences can be implemented simultaneously to incorporate these and other grammatical morphemes until all have been acquired. In each training sequence, the various constructions are presented several times at one level until an arbitrarily established criterion is met before moving to the next level. In addition, the child is reinforced when a particular goal is achieved (e.g., the seven-word, eight-morpheme combination Article + Noun + Auxiliary + Verb + ing + on + Article + Noun is the goal for level VIII). No other response would be acceptable. Within a relatively short time, the child may produce this seven-word, eight-morpheme combination, but most likely no grammatical forms other than those that were trained would be present in the child's speech. Those who have used this approach will probably agree that children do acquire the feature being trained. More times than not, however, the child performs these structures in a robot-like manner without any real understanding of their form or usage.

The goal of the horizontal developmental approach is the same as that of the vertical approach, but the method of approach gives the child a little more latitude for communication purposes. Normal children do not complete the acquisition of one linguistic construction (e.g., grammatical morphemes) before beginning to acquire another linguistic construction (e.g., pronouns). Instead, several linguistic constructions are simultaneously acquired at each developmental level. The horizontal developmental approach involves training a multitude of linguistic elements at a particular mean length of utterance (MLU) level before moving on to a more advanced level for each element.

Perhaps an illustration will provide a clear understanding of this procedure. Let's consider a child at the 1.5 MLU level and say that we wish to advance to the 2.0–2.5 MLU level. A normal child at the 2.0–2.5 MLU level uses a variety of construction types. Generally these include such forms as *Verb + Noun, Noun + Verb, Adjective + Noun, my + Noun, in + Noun, Verb + me, Noun + Verb* particle, *I + Verb* particle, to name a few (see Ingram and Eisenson, 1972, for an in-depth description of construction types by MLU level). Using the horizontal approach, the clinician would teach a number of different construction types at the same MLU level. The following excerpt, taken from a teaching session in which the clinician and the child are playing with a large red ball, illustrates the clinician's input in the horizontal approach.

Verb + Noun	roll ball
Noun + Verb	ball bounce
Adjective + Noun	red ball
my + Noun	my ball
in + Noun	in lap
Verb + me	bounce me
Noun + verb particle	ball throw up
I + verb particle	I throw up

In the horizontal developmental approach, one picture or activity is used as the stimulus for training a variety of construction types. With this approach, the child has the opportunity to observe that several different verbal responses are acceptable for the same stimulus activity. In this way horizontal training provides a natural situation for language learning. For this reason many clinicians choose the horizontal developmental approach over the vertical developmental approach.

PACKAGED PROGRAMS

The second instructional technique that makes use of the stimulus-response paradigm involves packaged programs. The salient feature of this technique is that it provides a rigid, preplanned, systematic approach to the acquisition of language. The child is led, step-by-step through the levels that the program authors feel are necessary for reaching a goal of appropriate language usage. Through various steps in the procedures, reinforcement techniques are utilized to increase the probability that a particular feature being trained will occur again.

What we find then, in these and other stimulus-response models, is that the child is provided with a good language model, is led through various developmental stages, and ultimately reaches his or her goal of adequate expressive form and function. Thus, the stimulus-response models are successful in helping language delayed children acquire linguistic structures that are absent from their speech.

We are finding, however, that when all is said and done, and the child is using adequate linguistic structure through whatever method, there is still something different about the child's use of language. That is, young language delayed children who proceed into the school setting continue to have language based problems. Inspection of structure and function indicates adequate performance. The children may even perform within the normal range on most traditional tests of language comprehension. However, they perform poorly on conceptual tests.

Whereas before we talked of grammatical morpheme deficiencies, semantic problems, and structural deficits, we now turn to language performance in the area of pragmatics. We notice that some children have difficulty with the communicative use of language. They have difficulty with conversational postulates, they don't know how to respond to questions or ask them, or how to use synonyms, antonyms, idioms, and metaphors. Is this inability to use language in a communicatively appropriate way the result of a language delay that has persisted, or is it a function of the methods that were used to remediate structural deficiencies? Probably, it is a combination of both. It is disheartening, however, to think that early intervention may be contributing to the problem.

We are told that early intervention with language delayed children gives them the best possible chance for success. Are we to throw away all that we have learned and believed to be true? One good point is that many school age children who show these communicative difficulties have never had early language remediation. For this reason I don't think that speech-language pathologists should feel that our intervention techniques are the sole cause of the problem. What we should be attentive to is the possibility that many of the young children we see may ultimately present us with these characteristics. It only makes sense then, to use early intervention techniques that promote good language, but at the same time incorporate abstract thinking. In other words, the more naturalness, and the less concreteness, the better the chance that some of the problems children have with abstract thinking may be aborted.

How can we modify our "standard" intervention techniques to try to incorporate some form of naturalness into the treatment session? Earlier I mentioned various forms of reinforcement and stated that many clinicians choose to use praise, tokens, and edible reinforcement. Meline (1980) has stated that there is a "continuum of naturalness" that can be used for reinforcement and that the appropriate response is the most natural form of reinforcement, then praise, then manipulation of objects, then tokens, the most unnatural being the use of food. Meline argued that we should design treatment techniques that are more "ecologically valid" by analyzing the "child's natural environment and using natural contingencies." I could not agree more. In the home environment, how many parents of normal children use edibles to teach their child to use various linguistic structures? The mere fact that children receive what is requested (Meline's appropriate response) should provide reinforcement enough for them to use a particular linguistic structure again. If we want to continue to use the stimulus-response type of model, we should at least use the most natural forms of reinforcement possible. In other words, we can modify stimulus-response techniques by altering the consequent event to a more natural form.

Another naturalness issue associated with stimulus-response intervention techniques is what the clinician is going to accept as a correct response from the child. For example, if the training goal is to teach the auxiliary *is*, treatment could take the following form. The clinician presents a picture of a man sitting at a table eating. The clinician says "What's the man doing?" The child responds "Eating." The clinician then says "No, the man *is* eating; say 'The man *is* eating.'" The child then says "The man is eating" and receives whatever form of reinforcement is being used.

The child soon learns that reinforcement can be received by responding with an Article + Noun + Auxiliary + Verb + ing type of response and is on the way to achieving yet another goal of language training. Through close inspection, however, one can see that the child's original response ("Eating") was, by adult standards, well within the acceptable range of discourse. What has occurred then, is the "training out," if you will, of the adult ellipsis discourse rule and the "training in" of the notion that completeness equals correctness. In the natural sense, we have led the child astray. We all use this discourse rule of ellipsis in normal conversation. Why then must we insist that a language delayed child be forced into an unnatural response? We should therefore preserve naturalness by allowing the child some flexibility in responding to a verbal stimulus. Wherever possible, we should accept elliptical responses. For similar reasons, we should also use open ended stimulus questions as much as possible. That is, suppose I say "What is the lady doing?" while presenting a picture of a lady sitting in a chair reading a book. One correct response is "Reading," for it fits the discourse rule and is the most salient feature in the picture. If the child says "Sitting," he or she still has met the criterion of correctness, even though this is an unusual response, because the question can be answered by a specific one-word response. Now, presenting the same picture to the child, I say "Tell me what's happening." This time the response "Sitting" is no longer correct. An utterance longer that one word is necessary for the discourse unit to be correct.

PARENT-CHILD INTERACTIONS AND USES OF PLAY

Thus far I have discussed reinforcement techniques, discourse rules and question types, and how they should be incorporated into language training to try to achieve naturalness. Still another aspect of concern comes from parent-child interaction studies, which have shown that parents who are "nondirective" tend to have children who respond better. When parents of normal and language delayed children are compared, parents of language disordered children do more commanding, demanding, requesting, asking, and labeling than do parents of normal children. Yet we give the language delayed child more of the same in the clinical situation by using the stimulus-response technique. Why do we take a "directive" approach in remediation?

To utilize a nondirective approach in training, we must replace the stimulus-response model by one that emphasizes various forms of "play." Most people who have argued against play as a viable clinical technique have done so because play seems to lack structure. Granted, no derivative of play could ever approach the structure and organization of stimulus-response training.

The focus of attention when initiating treatment by means of play is what the child is doing and saying. The clinician can still question. The clinician can still reinforce verbal responses by performing the act requested by the child, whether the verbalization is elliptical or complete. Here the child is controlling the antecedent event rather than the clinician, although the clinician can encourage the use of particular linguistic constructions by selecting topics for training, structuring input, and utilizing expansions. Parents of normal children informally use expansions to maintain or clarify the semantic intent of an utterance. Thus, when the language delayed child is reinforced for an elliptical response, the clinician should expand the utterance, keeping the semantic intent of the child's message, and should include linguistic constructions that are in need of remediation. Hence, we have a "structured play" treatment session that resembles a natural language learning environment. Currently we are seeing a revitalization of "play therapy" techniques that incorporate many of the same issues discussed here (Blodgett and Miller, 1981; Newhoff and Wilcox, 1981).

CONCLUSION

All of us at some time or another have wondered what becomes of the young language delayed child when he or she reaches school age. Will the child be enrolled in a normal classroom? Will the child be able to function in the classroom? Will the child always have difficulty with the pragmatic aspects of speech? These are important questions that we should attend to while the child is still young. Wouldn't it be nice to say that we have not only remediated the language problem of a child, but have paved the way for his or her future academic success? By continuing to modify language training approaches as we understand more about the language development of normal children, someday we will meet this goal.

REFERENCES

Blodgett, E. G., and Miller, V. P. 1981. The facilitative language model. Miniseminar presented at the American Speech-Language and Hearing Association Convention, Los Angeles.

Brown, R. 1973. A First Language, The Early Stages. Harvard University Press, Cambridge, Mass.

Ingram, D., and Eisenson, J. 1972. Therapeutic approaches in congenitally aphasic children. In: J. Eisenson (ed.), Aphasia in Children. Harper & Row, New York.

Hubbell, RD 1981   Children's Language Disorders: An Integrated Approach, Prentice Hall, Engleman PP 42-69

Meline, T. J. 1980. The application of reinforcement in language intervention. Lang. Speech Hear. Serv. Schools 11:95–101.

Newhoff, M., and Wilcox. M. J. 1981. Language intervention from a socio-communicative perspective. Short course presented at the American Speech-Language and Hearing Association Convention, Los Angeles.

Steckol, Karen F.

CHAPTER 2

Data Based Language Programs
A Closer Look

Kyla Becker Marion

Marion critically reviews "data based" language programs. Her critique poses some important questions about current language teaching principles.

1. *Marion speaks of "data based" language programs. What does this term mean? In what way has account-ability influenced the development of data based language programs?*
2. *In some language teaching approaches a task analysis is used. Define this tool. One objective of a task analysis is errorless learning. Do you believe this concept can be usefully applied to language teaching? What are some other objectives of a task analysis?*
3. *How may excessive record keeping interfere with language learning? Do you subscribe to the principle that frequent evaluation of language performance is important? If you do, what kind of ongoing evaluations do you recommend?*

PUBLIC LAW 94-142, THE EDUCATION FOR ALL HANDICAPPED CHILDREN ACT, mandates that a free and appropriate education be provided for all handicapped children between the ages of 5 and 21 years. The law further requires the development of an individualized education program (IEP), which includes written educational plans at the beginning of each school year, annual goals, and short-term instructional objectives written in behavioral terms by the instructor. Some IEPs also include a description of the method used to evaluate on a biannual basis the short-term objectives, the level of performance expected (criteria), and the expected date of completion. When appropriate, parents are invited to a planning conference to review and revise the individual plans. Placement agencies in most school districts must have on file an IEP for all children who receive special education services.

The desire to provide a quality education for all handicapped children is particularly evident in the field of speech and language. In accordance with PL 94-142, consent forms for all evaluative services must be on file before school clinicians may assess speech and language functions. In New York City, clinicians are required to use standardized assessment tools in their evaluations, and they must discuss in full all results and recommendations with parents at an educational planning conference. Because of strong government ties to special education, as well as the monetary issues involved, new demands for accountability are being proposed and implemented. A strong case for accountability was proposed by Caccamo (1973), who suggested that clinicians should not only predict the results of treatment, but should also guarantee some modicum of success. Caccamo called this "performance contracting." Some feel that a commitment to accountability ensures greater control and planning to procedures that in the past have been vague or ambiguous (Gerber, 1977). Legislators and administrators are demanding reports containing information on the productivity of individual intervention programs (McReynolds, 1974). Many states now require evidence of individualized short-term instructional objectives and quantification of treatment results before aid is allocated. Parents have become more vocal in their demands to review treatment goals, delivery systems, and periodic progress reports on their children.

Thus, speech and language clinicians in an attempt to satisfy IEP demands from federal and municipal agencies, supervisors, and parents, are having to seek speech and language procedures that contain in their administration and strategies for intervention the necessary ingredients for success. Often this pressure to be accountable may encourage the adoption, but not necessarily the adaptation, of enticingly packaged language programs filled with predetermined behavioral objectives, task analyses, data sheets for scoring and charting responses, criterion testing procedures, and specific guidelines for remediation. These programs stress individual instruction, refer to training rather than teaching, and emphasize achievement rather than intervention. In this chapter, language programs that contain a majority of these features are referred to as "data based."

Within the last decade, the cognitive, semantic, and pragmatic bases for language development have received considerable attention. Individuals who subscribe to these paradigms usually prefer intervention programs that are looser and less structured and have a more pronounced communicative basis. The student's desire to learn about the world and to interact with the environment provides the focal point for these more process oriented programs. Yet many knowledgable clinicians and administrators are purchasing and using data based language programs. In trying to obtain an effective intervention program that satisfies IEP guidelines, these professionals may be using data based language programs for the wrong reasons.

This chapter explores several issues related to data based language programs. First, we discuss factors contributing to the popularity of these programs. Second, we examine the effectiveness of data based language programs in the remediation of language disorders. Finally, we present guidelines for evaluating language programs in light of current research in language acquisition and remediation.

TRYING TO BE ACCOUNTABLE

Suppose as a clinician you are faced with the IEP commitment, the uncertainty of a supervisory visit, the eager anticipation of parents ready to review pretest and posttest scores and progress data, and a large heterogeneous caseload of language disordered children. How would you begin to resolve these pressures? Consider the following remarks made by speech and language pathologists when asked about their jobs. Do any of these statements sound familiar to you?

1. "I would like a predetermined, sequenced list of language behaviors."
2. "Planning individual lessons takes too much time."
3. "I want my students to learn as quickly as possible."
4. "My students should continually experience success."
5. "I want a language program I can use with all my students."
6. "I need activities that will ensure generalization of language behaviors trained in the clinic."

7. "I want some method of determining when my students have mastered a skill."
8. "Progress data should be available to parents when they meet with me to discuss their children."
9. "Progress data should be available to my supervisors when they meet with me to discuss my intervention strategies."
10. "I want to be accountable."

Program directors, curriculum writers, supervisors, and teacher trainers are aware of these issues as they evaluate and purchase language materials and programs for their clinics and schools. Budgetary considerations and the need for quick progress and discharge, to accommodate students on waiting lists, are additional factors felt by these specialists.

Catalogs and publications describing a variety of language programs are received almost daily by clinicians and administrators. Although publishers may offer little information regarding the rationale of their programs, they usually place great emphasis on the ability of these programs to satisfy IEP requirements. The stress on accountability is especially apparent in the descriptive paragraphs introducing data based language programs. These programs, responsive to the needs of the clinician, emphasize efficiency, universality, and economy. Data based language programs usually offer prewritten behavioral objectives, step-by-step task analysis of each objective, and a highly organized, carefully structured method of intervention. These programs usually indicate what to teach and often suggest how to teach it. It is not hard to understand why these programs have great appeal to the consumer interested in being accountable.

Data based language programs claim to provide a systematic, instructional system that meets federal and state guidelines. To accomplish this, programs are written that clearly satisfy the clinician's need for accountability but may ignore the unique and individual needs of the student. More attention may be given to testing and tracking than to teaching. When teaching activities are provided, they seem to be influenced more by programming and administrative concerns than by current research in the cognitive, semantic, and pragmatic areas. The clinician who utilizes these programs "as is" may be "looking good," but not "teaching good." Finally, data based language programs may contain certain elements harmful to the growth of language behaviors in children. This chapter explores and evaluates the following components, usually contained in data based language programs: task analysis, scoring procedures, extension activities for generalization, and the predetermined response.

TASK ANALYSIS: ERRORLESS LEARNING

Data based language programs usually provide a task analysis for each language objective to be trained. Task analysis refers to the method of dividing a behavior into small, manageable units. Each step in the series is built on the previous skill and depends on it. On paper, these highly structured steps may have great appeal for those who want a "cookbook" approach to treatment. However, a task analysis that works well for certain skill areas, such as sharpening a pencil or making a bed, may be far too linear, unidirectional, and simplistic for an activity as complex as using language. In addition, the way a task analysis is written may directly influence the choice of intervention strategies. For example, consider the following task analysis for the target behavior eye contact:

1. Looks in direction of trainer
2. Looks directly at trainer
3. Looks at face of trainer
4. Looks at eye of trainer

Prewritten sequences, like this illustration, are found in data based language programs that feature strong stimulus-response-consequence approaches to language teaching. The student is rewarded for the number of seconds of actual eye contact, but the communicative intent of the learner's response may be neither considered nor developed. The stress on behavior and the measurement of that behavior are of prime importance when one subscribes to this type of sequence. A better technique for facilitating eye contact might be to list the following precursors:

1. Uses clinician to satisfy physical needs
2. Uses clinician to gain attention
3. Uses clinician to obtain an object

With this list of prerequisite behaviors, strategies would be developed to create a need or desire in the student to perform a particular behavior, and to use the clinician as a means to satisfy this need or to achieve a goal. Eye contact would evolve naturally as a method of achieving contact and interaction with the clinician.

Data based language programs geared to the development of linguistic forms may also contain poorly designed task analyses. Consider the following example, where the task of producing an auxiliary "is" plus a present progressive is divided into a three-step sequence:

1. Jumping
2. Is jumping
3. Girl is jumping

In the next example, a two-constituent utterance is divided into its component parts:

1. Johnny
2. Name Johnny
3. My name Johnny

The behavioral strategy usually used to teach sequences like those illustrated above is called backward chaining. This technique may be an appropriate method for teaching a retarded child to make a bed (blanket, cover sheet, and bottom sheet); however, children simply do not learn morphologic and syntactical rule systems in this manner or sequence.

There are many reasons for the highly structured, but superficial, task analysis found in most data based language programs. Some program writers may not understand the process of normal language acquisition. In addition, many programmers believe that it is easier to monitor responses or to measure progress when the skills measured are small or discrete. Finally, many feel that by dividing a language behavior into smaller, more manageable steps, they can keep the proportion of correct responses high. Skinner (1969) said that programs should not allow for many errors because the best learning takes place when students make correct responses. He also suggested that producing correct responses motivates and intensifies the student's desire to work hard. This stress on errorless learning is questionable because most language learning occurs in a revisionist or trial-and-error fashion. The research literature is filled with many examples of children making "errors" on their way to acquiring adult forms. This desire on the part of some language clinicians to encourage errorless learning may result in data forms filled with correct responses without necessarily being in the best interest of the learner. When choosing a language program, clinicians should evaluate carefully the sequence of each task analysis, because the design of the sequence may well be in opposition to the normal acquisition of language.

MEASURING THE PRODUCT

Clinicians have recently been seeking language programs that include pretesting and posttesting procedures. Though data collection is not a new technique, responses have not usually been recorded daily in traditional language remediation. However, parents and administrators are now asking for quantification to prove that learning has occurred. Some feel that informal evaluations of language behaviors are based on arbitrary decisions or intuition rather than on scientific evidence (Mowrer, 1969). According to Mowrer, error rate profiles may provide useful information concerning the difficulty of the task and may lead to modifications of the task, the teaching strategies, or the learning environment. Although the need for recording student progress is recognized, the emphasis on keeping score in most data based language programs may be detrimental to the learning process insofar as it influences the way a clinician views training.

The focal point of a training session may be the scoring of responses rather than the facilitation of language learning. Little attention may be paid to the communicative intent of the utterance, the nonverbal message present, or the student's strategies for decoding language. Instead, more thought may be given to the careful arrangement of data sheets and score forms, as well as the accurate charting of responses. The pressure to record data continually during intervention is especially apparent when one uses a language program stressing a behavioral approach.

Data based language programs are usually designed to elicit language production rather than language processing because words are easier to score or chart than ideas or cognitive notions. For example, to learn the concept *under*, the student may be expected to respond correctly to the following series of questions:

> Q. *Where is the ball?* A. *Under the table.*
> Q. *Where is the doll?* A. *Under the bed.*
> Q. *Where is the pencil?* A. *Under the desk.*

The cognitive notions of space, and the relative position of an object in space, precursors to the locative *under*, may not be taught by clinicians because they may believe that these ideas cannot be measured easily in behavioral terms. Therefore, teaching may be ignored in favor of testing, and the language product, rather than the process of learning language, may become the goal of the lesson. However, correct performance on a task does not necessarily mean comprehension or integration of a rule system.

Many believe that objective data are necessary for recording the progress of a client to evaluate the effectiveness of an intervention strategy (Girardeau and Spradlin, 1970). Yet pretest and posttest data do not ensure a cause-and-effect relationship between progress and intervention. Data based language programs may claim such relationships, but usually they offer no real empirical evidence to support such claims.

GENERALIZING LANGUAGE BEHAVIORS

Most language programs suggest that the ultimate goal of training is the generalization of target vocabulary, morphemes, and syntactic structures in the natural environment of the child. According to traditional practices, the clinician usually provides for generalization by including a culminating activity and a homework assignment. Writers of data based program suggest that generalization can be obtained by using a procedure at the end of the training called the application activity or the extension acitivity. These procedures are designed to help individuals use newly acquired language behaviors in a variety of situations and settings.

These programs may also include forms for checking both generalization and long-term maintenance of trained behaviors. Generalization is sought in the clinical setting, the classroom, during free play, or at home. To determine whether claims of generalization by data based language programs can be realized, the concept of generalization should be defined. According to Skinner (1957), generalization has occurred if a behavior conditioned in the presence of a particular stimulus or situation is observed more readily in the presence of a stimulus showing properties similar to those of the first. Most program writers would agree that generalization is more likely to occur when there is similarity between the training environment and the real world, yet few provisions are made to create this similarity in most highly structured language programs.

Data based language programs are strikingly alike in their strategies for achieving generalization of language behaviors. Many programmers feel that language disordered children cannot extract meaning or linguistic structures from their natural environment (Gray and Fygetakis, 1968). Thus, data based language programs often begin by isolating and training a target behavior in a controlled, sterile, and quiet environment, void of paralinguistic cues. Many programs screen out the "noise" and concentrate on either a stimulus-response method or the drilling, repetition, or modeling of various linguistic patterns.

Generalization is often treated as a separate issue and is provided for later in the training, as a child is presented with similar stimuli or settings in a more naturalistic environment. Often a classroom teacher or a parent is asked to present the stimulus to ensure that generalization has occurred across individuals as well as across settings. However, if one subscribes to the philosophy that language behaviors are more likely to generalize if they are originally facilitated in a communicatively rich environment, the training session appears to be upside down.

The culminating activity or extension procedure should occur *first*, not *last*. For example, the morpheme *ing* should be facilitated in an environment where actions are talked about as they are performed; to enable this language form to be associated both with meaning and with communicative intent. Most data based programs train the *ing* separately, using patterned drill, and then test for the generalization of this morpheme in free play.

Another example may help illustrate this point. A child who is learning to include the subject in a three-constituent utterance is often drilled with dozens of action pictures illustrating subject, verb, and object complement. The student may be expected to repeat the following pattern:

The boy is breaking the truck.
The girl is hitting the ball.
The dog is eating the bone.

Generalization training may be provided for later in free play by showing the child similar pictures and asking the question, "What is happening in the picture?" An alternative approach might be an action game requiring turn taking. Each student must describe what his or her partner is doing before taking a turn performing an action. The students must use the first name of their partners when describing the action. For example:

Susan is clapping her hands.
Mario is scratching his head.
Chi is snapping his fingers.
Davida is touching her toes.

Here the subject is the first constituent in a three-constituent utterance. The student does not learn nor subsequently generalize the subject by repeating patterns out of context. The use of the subject is based on the knowledge that to be understood in a communicatively based activity, the subject must be marked clearly as a referent.

In summary, language behaviors must originate in a meaningful environment if language learners are to generalize those behaviors to other contexts, on their own. Ironically, in most data based programs, the opposite occurs. The child experiences the target behavior in isolation and is then expected to show evidence of having learned the behavior in a new context or situation in the last 10 minutes of a clinical session. Have some language programs put the cart before the horse?

PREPROGRAMMED RESPONSES

In traditional language programming, clinicians usually identify the behaviors that should be facilitated to reach the objective or terminal goal of the lesson. During the interaction, the clinician must then decide whether a student's response is appropriate to the task. These decisions should be made by analyzing the semantic content of the utterance, the syntactic and morphological aspects, and the communicative intent of the speaker. The clinician then has the option of reinforcing, commenting on, correcting, or ignoring the response. Data based language programs make these decisions for the clinician. That is, they determine a priori the desired response. Decisions of this kind are usually based on the rationale or model of language training that is built into the program. Acceptable responses may reflect the semantic, linguistic, or pragmatic interest of the program writer. Most data based language programs appear to accept only one response for each stimulus. All responses are then judged right or wrong accordingly. A correct response is usually an exact duplication of the answer written into the program or found on the response sheet.

The foregoing discussion of the preprogramming of correct responses raises two important questions:

1.   Can we predict responses made by children acquiring language?
2.   Should we preprogram these responses?

Based on a variety of clinical experiences with language learners, most clinicians would probably agree that we cannot predetermine exactly how a child will respond to each stimulus in a program. Children may produce a variety of responses to a given stimulus (Blank, 1978). For example, if you hold up a square and ask for the name, responses may include "box," "rectangle," and "yellow." Although these answers may not be found on the program's response sheet, they may reflect a learner's individual strategy in processing the stimulus. A child who has a retrieval problem may answer with a categorical response (rectangle), whereas another may have just received a classroom lesson on the color yellow. Nelson (1977) believes that one of the most important characteristics of early language behaviors consists of the multitude of errors children make in their struggle to create new sentences. Because the language of children often has rule systems different from the language of adults, and because the strategies children use to acquire language are not always the same, it seems impossible to predict exact responses and unfair to program them. In an effort to create a universal language program, some data based programs expect more consistency than most children evidence in their efforts to learn language. Although programmers may have a particular response in mind, they should consider a wide range of possible verbal behaviors. The learner should not be forced or pushed into responding in a "predictable" way. The programmer, not the client, may need to adapt.

"INCORRECT" RESPONSES

Since most data based language programs place great emphasis on the daily monitoring of correct/incorrect answers, this monitoring procedure is examined in more detail. The recording of a correct response and its consequence may not present a problem for the student. Most children like to receive praise and to collect tokens redeemable for prizes. However, it is necessary to examine procedures dealing with "incorrect responses" for at least two reasons.

1. One consequence of an "incorrect response" may be to reduce the utilization of verbal behavior by a child.
2. We may be penalizing our students for using their own acquisitional strategies in responding to a stimulus.

In a study some years ago, Lovaas (1968) suggested that incorrect verbal behavior should not be punished. Most programmers agree with Lovaas and simply ignore and/or record incorrect responses. However, ignoring a student's language behavior, or placing a 0 instead of an X on a data sheet may be punishing. Children know when positive reinforcement of feedback has been omitted. Such omissions may inhibit the learner's spontaneity, end the desire to take risks, and act to limit other verbal behaviors.

Some data based language programs do not permit individual strategies either in the processing or in the production of language. For example, a student who is asked to describe a picture showing a boy running may say "Boy running." If the target behavior is to produce the auxiliary "is," the response may be judged to be "incorrect." Yet the learner is correct at the semantic level; he or she knows not only the lexical items, but the temporal concept of the present progressive. The student is also correct at the morphological level, because *ing* has been correctly produced. However, because this response is judged to be "incorrect," the student receives no social praise (reward). Moreover, the student may not be told why the response is considered incorrect.

Program writers who put great emphasis on prewritten responses should recognize that all aspects of language are operating at the same time even when an "error" is present. Just as we acknowledge that language behaviors should not be taught in isolation, we must also evaluate responses within the total communicative framework. All language programs should incorporate a strategy for accepting a student's utterance on some level, even though the student has failed to produce the target response. The clinician's knowledge of normal language acquisition will help to determine the proper feedback when errors are made.

EVALUATING LANGUAGE PROGRAMS

There are probably more than 250 language programs, many of them data based, available commercially or published in journals and textbooks. Guidelines for evaluating these programs usually deal with programming issues such as reinforcement scheduling, reward systems, and criterion levels, rather than the more critical issues raised in this chapter. In addition, many of the programs remain untested. There is a need for guidelines to use in evaluating these programs. It is suggested that clinicians ask the following questions when assessing a language program:

1. How does the program define language?
2. What aspects of language does the program claim to develop?
3. What model or models of language intervention does the program advocate?
4. Does the program follow the normal development of language in planning assessment and intervention strategies?
5. What assessment procedures were used to determine placement in the program?
6. Are the assessment procedures adequate in determining the student's present level of performance?
7. For what population is the program designed?
8. Can the program be used for group as well as individual instruction?
9. Does the program establish language concepts through comprehension as well as expression?
10. Are the lessons taught in a communicative, transactional environment?
11. What procedures are used to create generalization of language behaviors?
12. Does the program predetermine behavioral objectives, task analysis, and response modes?
13. How does the program allow for the individual differences of the students?
14. How does the program allow for "errors"?
15. Are the materials salient, age appropriate, and of interest to the child?
16. What data are available on the validity of the program?
17. Who has reviewed this program and what has been said?
18. If you had the time to develop individual behavioral objectives

and intervention strategies for all your students, would you still use this program?

BEING ACCOUNTABLE IN THE 1980s: A POSTSCRIPT

A review of the current literature on language programs reveals a striking absence of critical evaluation and research. Program writers describe, evaluate, and applaud their own approaches, but school systems and clinics, although they purchase and use these programs, usually fail to note any problems or to question the effectiveness of data based language programs. Some professionals appear to view these programs not as models worthy of discussion, but as a quick way of satisfying their commitment to accountability and the IEP. But this chapter has suggested that our commitment to our students and their individual differences and strategies for learning language (a rationale for IEP development) may be ignored by such programs.

Current research in language acquisition and intervention appears to be taking one direction, while language programs that promise accountability may be taking another. Thus, clinicians may find themselves in a state of conflict as they strive to be both accountable and current. The IEP does not create the problem; this document does not tell us what to teach or how to teach it. The choice remains with the clinician. Being truly accountable in the 1980s means adopting intervention strategies that emanate from basic research and recognize the individuality of the learner. If language programs are used, they should satisfy the student's need, not the clinician's. One does not need scores of data sheets to convince parents that their children have made progress. Being accountable in the 1980s may mean more work for the clinician, but better learning for the student.

REFERENCES

Blank, M. 1978. A communication model for assessing and treating language disorders. Paper presented at the Nato International Conference on Rehabilitation of Learning Disorders, Quebec, June 1978.

Caccamo, J. M. 1973. Accountability—A matter of ethics? Asha 15:411–412.

Gerber, A. 1977. Programming for articulation modification. J. Speech Hear Disord. 42:29–43.

Girardeau, F. L., and Spradlin, J. E. 1970. An introduction to the functional analysis of speech and language. In: F. L. Girardeau and J. E. Spradlin (eds.), A Functional Analysis Approach to Speech and Language. Asha Monogr. 14:1–9.

Gray, B., and Fygetakis, L. 1968. Mediated language acquisition for dyphasic children. Behav. Res. Ther. 6:263–280.

Lovaas, O. I. 1968. A program for the establishment of speech in psychotic children. In: H. N. Sloane and B. D. MacAulay (eds.), Operant Procedures in Remedial Speech and Language Training, pp. 125–154 Houghton-Mifflin, Boston.

McReynolds, L. V. 1974. Introduction to developing systematic procedures. In: L. V. McReynolds (ed.), Developing Systematic Procedures for Training Children's Language. Asha Monogr. 18:1–4.

Mowrer, D. E. 1969. Evaluating speech therapy through precision recording. J. Speech Hear. Dis. 34:239–244.

Nelson, K. E. 1977. Aspects of language acquisition and use from age 2 to age 20. J. Am. Acad. Child Psychiatry 16:584–607.

Skinner, B. F. 1957. Verbal Behavior. Appleton-Century-Crofts, New York.

Skinner, B. F. 1969. Contingencies of Reinforcement: A Theoretical Analysis. Appleton-Century-Crofts, New York.

CHAPTER 3

Use and Abuse of the Developmental Approach

Harris Winitz

In his evaluation of the developmental model of language teaching, Winitz contrasts this method of instruction with an approach that emphasizes comprehension and nonlinear teaching, for which he details a number of language intervention procedures.

1. *According to Winitz, there are three major premises that underlie the developmental model of language teaching. Rephrase each premise in your own terms.*
2. *What flaws in the developmental model of language teaching are revealed by the study of children's errors in language development? Furthermore, on what basis does this model prescribe procedures for providing language input? Do you agree with this approach?*
3. *What is meant by the statement, "Language stages represent outcomes or accomplishments, but not language processes"? How are accomplishments interpreted in the developmental model of language teaching? Why does Winitz disagree with this interpretation?*
4. *Contrast linear and nonlinear language learning. What evidence seems to argue against linear learning as a model for language instruction?*
5. *Distinguish between "forced production" and "encouraging speech through communication." What theoretical differences separate these two approaches?*
6. *Describe the clinical procedure identified as "goal directed activity." What is the theoretical basis for this approach? Do you agree that this method is appropriate for teaching language?*

A WELL-ESTABLISHED REMEDIAL MODEL in language training involves the use of developmental stages to formulate the content of language training programs (Crystal, Fletcher, and Garman, 1976; Miller and Yoder, 1974; Prutting, 1979). This model of language training has come to be called the developmental approach.

Clinicians have offered differing approaches for the treatment of delayed language within the developmental framework. However, these differences are largely differences of detail, encompassing such issues as which words to teach first (Holland, 1975; Lahey and Bloom, 1977), which grammatical structures to emphasize (Crystal et al., 1976), which activities (modeling, imitation, etc.) to use for implementing the language program, and how to provide a proper balance between the teaching of communicative functions and grammatical structures (McLean and Snyder-McLean, 1978). These differences do not impair the underlying framework of the developmental approach. It is a highly accepted clinical model, deeply a part of the teaching tradition of most speech and language pathologists.

What is the basis for the developmental approach? A major consideration is that language-delayed children should be taught to acquire the form, content, and function of language in essentially the same order that normal children acquire language. Additionally, the language teaching routines are to simulate, as closely as possible, the factors that contribute to normal language development. I take the position that the developmental model of language teaching is, in principle, basically sound. Yet I also suggest that it is generally used incorrectly, and, for this reason, its effectiveness as an intervention model may not be properly realized.

DEVELOPMENTAL MODEL: SOME PREMISES

The first step in treatment is to examine thoroughly the language performance of each child before developing a plan for language training. Of course, diagnosis and assessment continue throughout the training program to provide flexibility in the treatment plan. One procedure is to establish a language age for each child. For example, a child who is 4 years old, but utters only two-word responses is equivalent in syntactic development to an 18-month to 24-month-old child.

Some children with delayed language exhibit deficiencies that extend across several language age levels. In these cases an age level equivalent is not particularly meaningful. For purposes of treatment the clinician will note the lowest age level at which there is a language deficiency and begin training at that developmental level (Miller and Yoder, 1974; Prutting, 1979).

This premise is one of three basic premises of the developmental approach. Restated, premise 1 is expressed as follows.

PREMISE 1   Establish the lowest language level according to developmental norms at which a language deficiency occurs, and begin teaching at that level.

There are a number of other premises that follow from the first. One pertains to the criteria that are used to discontinue training at one developmental level and to begin training at the next higher level. A common approach is not to begin training at the next higher developmental level until all language elements for a particular level have been acquired. This is, premise 2, stated as follows.

PREMISE 2   The elements targeted for training within a language age level should be acquired by the child before training is begun at the next higher developmental level of language.

A third premise of training, which is associated with the first two, involves a generally accepted procedural goal of language training. Usually clinicians gauge performance in language learning by success in speaking. This measure of performance seems to be intuitively correct and that is why it is often stressed. Holland (1975, pp. 517–518) exemplified this position in her description of the practices of an individual whom she referred to as a model language clinician. "I observed a therapy session in which a gifted clinician was teaching *more*. She. . .had plans eventually to demand the word from the child." In this particular example, as so often is the case, a fundamental objective in language teaching is to define achievement in terms of language production. When this criterion of language achivement is applied to the developmental model, it means that language instruction is to be restricted to a developmental language level until the form, content, and function for that level have been acquired as an expressive skill. Premise 3 emphasizes production.

PREMISE 3   Successful language achievement is indicated by the ability to produce or express language through speech. For this reason, language training is to be restricted to a developmental language level until achievement is demonstrated by correct usage in production of that level for all language elements.

Of course, when it has been determined that speech is not possible, other forms of production such as sign language, writing, or other systems of nonverbal communication may be taught. These alternatives are not addressed in this chapter.

Thus according to the three basic premises of the developmental approach to language teaching, training should begin at the lowest level at which there is a deficiency and should be continued at that level until mastery in production is achieved before going on to the next higher level.

Now let us challenge each of these three premises. Although each is intuitively appealing, each is counter to our understanding of how language is acquired by children under natural circumstances. The possibility that these three premises may not be in accord with how language is learned by normally developing children is not sufficient reason for their rejection. It is possible that procedures of teaching can emphasize processes markedly different from those that are inferred to be the case in the development of language, and at the same time may be effective and useful. However, the premises cited above have been offered as useful guidelines largely on the belief that they reflect normal language processes. As teaching routines, they are said to be directly supported by research in normal language development. We will show that this interpretation is not the case and that, furthermore, the implementation of these premises probably retards the growth of language. Additionally, there is no independent evidence to support these premises. There are, for example, no clinical studies demonstrating that implementation of the three premises will teach language. In fact, substantive comparative studies of language teaching methods are not available.

LANGUAGE ACQUISITION

Most language theorists contend that children formulate hypotheses about the patterned language input that they hear. For this reason language acquisition is regarded to be an active rather than a passive process. These hypotheses or theories are not necessarily consciously available to the language learner. Nonetheless, they provide the underlying framework for the task of language processing.

As children acquire language, they are engaged in sifting through large amounts of language data (language input) to understand their meaning with reference to the situation in which the data occur as utterances. Older children learning a second language are able to express this very point. For example, 13-year-old Ricardo was asked in Spanish what he did to process the English he heard; Butterworh and

Hatch (1978, p. 235) reported that "He listened for a few key words. He applied what he could understand to the immediate context and responded appropriately."

One strategy of Ricardo was to focus on the meaning of the language. A strategy is a method for solving problems. The strategies that children formulate are both linguistic and nonlinguistic. For example, young children often apply a strategy in which the first noun in a sentence is regarded as the agent, the performer of the activity. This strategy works well as a linguistic hypothesis for most sentence types that young children hear, but, of course, will cause difficulty in understanding passive sentences, such as "The boy was helped by the girl." If *boy* is interpreted as agent, the sentence will be incorrectly interpreted to mean "The boy helped the girl."

A number of early language learning strategies has been outlined by Chapman (1978). As she indicated, one strategy that children use is to act on objects that are visible or the center of attention. For example, a child standing in front of a chair will sit down on the chair when given the verbal command "sit down" accompanied by the appropriate gesture. The child may not understand this verbal command but can infer its meaning from contextual cues and the physical prominence of the chair. Another strategy young children use is to perform according to the way things are usually done. If told to put the spoon under the bowl, they will most likely place it in the bowl because spoons are usually placed there. In short, children develop and utilize certain strategies, linguistic and nonlinguistic, to extract the communicative meaning of utterances addressed to them. These strategies, of course, change as the children develop increased sophistication about language.

Errors that children make are often believed to be indicative of their underlying hypotheses about language. For example, a child who says *swinged* for *swung* or *buyed* for *bought* may have developed the theory that the past tense is always formed by adding the suffix "ed."

As children acquire additional knowledge about their language, they sometimes make errors they had not made before. For example, Bowerman (1978a) reported the illustrative utterance of a young child who had been told that she must go to bed. "I don't want to go to bed yet. Don't *let* me go to bed." The substitution error of *let* for *make* is interpreted as indicative of increased knowledge of these two verbs. Bowerman reasoned that the semantic properties of these verbs become similar as additional knowledge about them is acquired. This increase in similarity can cause errors. Analysis of children's errors, then, can tell us about the knowledge children implicitly hold about language.

The traditional methods that are used to measure children's knowledge of language for the purposes of designing a program of clinical instruction do not usually include an analysis of language errors. Language tests are largely based on correct usage, and in this regard they measure language achievement. These tests do not measure the formulation of language hypotheses. When the results of these tests are used to provide descriptive statements about language development, they indicate stages of language achievement, but not stages of language formulation. They provide only a passive overview of an active developmental process.

Additionally, measures of achievement are often limited to expressive language. It is now recognized that children comprehend more than they use in speech even when context is taken into account. For example, children who make two-word utterances have an understanding of language that goes beyond two-word sentences. Bloom (1970) noted, for example, that for one child the words "Wendy elevator" meant "Did Wendy come on the elevator?" and the utterance "Mommy pigtail" indicated "Mommy make me a pigtail." The contextual circumstances in which these two-word utterances occurred indicated that this child's understanding of language was greater than was evidenced by her use of two-word constructions. This inference is supported by the occurrence of two-word utterances that were rephrased by the child. For example, on one occasion Bloom's young subject said "Baby milk" (touching her mother's milk glass). Her mother responded "Baby's milk," and the child said "Touch milk," an indication that "touch" was implied in the original utterance "Baby milk." The child had meant to say "Baby touch milk." Performance constraint(s) apparently precluded a three-word utterance at this time, although the child comprehended three-word utterances and occasionally used them. Unfortunately, the developmental norms on which clinical language programs of instruction are based do not take this kind of information into account. Their focus is on performance levels of achievement, not on underlying processes.

INPUT IN LANGUAGE TRAINING

With these considerations in mind, it is constructive to reexamine premise 1. For example, children 4 years of age who use only one-word utterances are regarded as considerably delayed in language acquisition. According to premise 1, language teaching would begin at the next higher level. The goal would be to elicit two-word utterances from the children. This approach, advised by a number of clinicians (Lahey and Bloom, 1977; Miller and Yoder, 1974; Prutting, 1979), does not clearly specify the form of the language input that is presented to the language delayed child.

One recommendation is that the child be spoken to in two-word utterances (Miller and Yoder, 1974). However, it is difficult to use only two-word utterances and at the same time provide the child with realistic, communicative experiences. A variation of this approach is to use short, grammatically correct sentences more than two words long, but not to demand from the child utterances of more than two words. The clinician might say "Yes. I'll find the ball. Now you say 'the ball'; say '*the ball*.'" Or the clinician might use a question rather than a command to elicit an utterance. "Do you want the ball? Do you want the big ball or the small ball? Say '*small ball*.'" These are typical intervention strategies that are used to motivate children to talk.

The models of language intervention described above restrict the level of language input to the language stage directly above the child's level of functioning. However, this procedure effectively eliminates the use of pragmatically appropriate language, and in this regard differs from the normal circumstances that surround the development of language.

DEVELOPMENTAL STAGES ARE OUTCOMES

The developmental model of language instruction is largely based on the premise that the acquisition of language consists of stages of expressive language development as they have been observed to occur in the normally developing child. On the contrary, the evidence, as we have indicated, shows that children have receptive knowledge at various levels of development as they are acquiring the language. Also, at each developmental stage their language production generally is not restricted to that stage, nor can these structures be regarded as formulaic expressions (Brown, 1973). Rather, they are expressions that do not yet appear with enough consistency to be regarded as mastered, especially when the criterion level (often 90%) is high.

It is true that children progress from relatively simple utterances to complex and interesting language patterns. In this sense the developmental sequence is not a fiction. However, at any point in development the influence of succeeding stages is clearly indicated. Only, perhaps, in the very early stage of single-word development may children be operating within a clearly defined level. In all the other stages of development, children's verbal utterances contain instances of form, content, and function that are mastered at later age levels. For example, three-word sequences occasionally are used during the two-word stage. Also, morphological forms that are reported to develop relatively late are used with a certain degree of frequency at early age levels (Brown, 1973). Developmental stages, then, reflect age points at which mastery has been achieved, but do not indicate successive points in a learning sequence. Stated in another way, developmental stages are outcomes of a set of complex learning processes.

An analogy at this point may prove helpful. Suppose you are taking a foreign language course using a textbook that contains 40 chapters. Each chapter explains one or two grammatical principles. Your instructor tells you that you are to master each chapter before tackling the next one. You try to learn this way, but you often find that you are unable to integrate correctly some of the material learned in earlier chapters when trying to master later chapters. You also find, however, that some of the principles presented in later chapters provide explanation of material that was unclear when first presented in earlier chapters.

This procedure of learning in which one is to master a prescribed set of lessons in successive stages has been called *linear learning* (Winitz, 1981a). It is linear in the sense that learning is conceived as a straight line function beginning at one point and ending at another point. This particular learning style characterizes the developmental approach to language teaching. It says, in effect, that a child is to acquire language according to an orderly and prescribed sequence, as determined by the language stages of the normally developing child.

Language learning does not seem to work this way. Language learning is largely a nonlinear process. The input that a child receives is varied in complexity. Not all is understood at first, largely because all the information cannot be processed initially. However, there are other reasons. One is that each of the parts of language relates to every other part in complex and interlocking ways. Verb rules, for example, cannot be acquired without extensive exposure to many verbs, the contexts in which they are used, and the way in which verbs relate to other grammatical components. For example, verb conjugation rules alone will not explain the ungrammatical usage of the verbs *knowing* and *was* in the respective utterances "I am knowing" and "A cat was a pet."

The complex relationship among the component parts of language is illustrated in a report by Bowerman (1978b) on causative verbs, that is, verbs that are used in the sense of causing an event to take place, as in "She *closed* the door" (caused the door to be closed) or "He *cut* the meat" (caused the meat to be cut). Transitive verbs like *close* and *cut* can be used without modification to express causal relationships. Intransitive verbs, such as *die* and *sing*, require a change in form (*I killed him* for *I made him die*) or the use of certain verbs like *make*, as in *I made him sing* for the unallowable *I sang him*. Certain adjectives have different forms from their corresponding transitive verbs, such as *flat* and *flatten*, as in *I flatten the box*, or *full* and *fill*, as in *I filled it up*.

Bowerman provides examples of intransitive verbs and adjectives that initially were used correctly by children but later were used incorrectly in the expression of causal relationships. An example in which the adjective *full* was used incorrectly is the following utterance of a child a little more than 2 years of age: "*Full* it up" (fill up a bottle), and one in which the intransitive verb *come* was used incorrectly: "I *come* it closer so it won't fall" (meaning *make a bowl "come" closer* or more correctly, *bring the bowl closer to me*). On the surface it would appear that the child had not yet mastered the distinction between transitive verbs (those that take an object) and intransitive verbs (those that do not take an object) or between verbs and adjectives. In all likelihood, this child had acquired most recently a deep understanding of the English verb rule for expressing causal relationships, but incorrectly applies it to some adjectives and intransitive verbs in their unmodified form to be used as transitive verbs with causal intent.

In the developmental model of language teaching, as indicated above, achievement is defined as correct usage, usually 90–100% correct performance. If the developmental model of language teaching is strictly adhered to, it would place language clinicians in the difficult position of not being able to teach or provide as input a large number of verbs and adjectives before the stage at which causative verbs are correctly mastered. No one would, of course, suggest this course of action. Causative verbs need to be taught early largely because they express a fundamental relationship that cannot be avoided in communication.

Similarly it would not seem to be good clinical practice to organize the teaching of other language forms according to achievement levels. This does not mean that developmental language profiles should be totally ignored: they can serve as a guide for the *emphasis* of certain structures and, perhaps, the avoidance of others. However, these profiles should not be used as a fixed set of sequences from which the clinician cannot deviate.

The foregoing remarks demonstrate that premise 1, which emphasizes that training should be directed to the next level beyond a child's current level of language functioning, is not only impractical but unrealistic. It precludes the use of communicative centered language and speech training, and places both the child and the clinician in the uncomfortable position of talking about a restricted set of circumstances, just as we might visualize a college student who tries to create dialogues in French in the first week of the course or, for that matter, at the conclusion of the first semester. Meaningful dialogue is difficult when the use of language functions and structures is put under external, artificial constraints.

A variation of this position, as indicated above, is to restrict expressive language training to a single developmental level while providing input that extends beyond this level. This approach is a compromise that adds a degree of flexibility in the application of premises 1 and 2.

Premise 2, which is closely related to premise 1, states that there should be mastery of the language structures at each developmental level before the teaching of structures at the next higher level begins. As we have discussed, this approach is largely impractical and theoretically unsound. Language levels that are considerably more advanced than the next immediately higher level contribute importantly to knowledge at lower developmental levels. For example, of the 14 grammatical morphemes studied by Brown (1973), the present progressive suffix "ing" is acquired first [(e.g., The dog (is) eat*ing*.)] and considerably earlier than the morphemes for the third person singular, present tense (e.g., The dog eats), denoted here as [-s]. Yet it is unlikely that children are completely unaware of the semantic and grammatical implications of [-s] prior to the language stage at which achievement is demonstrated.

At this point it is not known with certainty why [-ing] develops before [-s]. Much has been written on the topic of order of acquisition, and many theories have been proposed that include factors relating to conceptual, semantic and/or linguistic complexity, input experience, articulatory constraints, innate tendencies, and so on. It is not possible to discuss all these interesting issues here. However, one point is mentioned. The [-s] is largely redundant because in the present tense, linguistic person is indicated by the pronoun (e.g., I eat, you eat, she/he/it eats, we eat, you eat, they eat). The contrast between the present and present progressive (e.g., He eats, he is eating; they eat, they are eating) is indicated by the presence or absence of [-ing], by the presence or absence of the auxiliaries "is" and "are," and redundantly by the [-s] for third person singular. No doubt the auxiliaries *is* and *are* are not salient initially for children, because they usually omit them when they first use the present progressive. Nor is the [-s] usually salient.

In some cases, such as for the frequent verbs *put*, *cut*, and *set*, the [-s] serves as a marker between past tense (he put, he cut, he set) and present tense (he puts, he cuts, he sets). It is of interest that [-s] develops after the regular past tense (Brown, 1973). No doubt there is a nonlinear effect here in that the addition of [-s] to present tense usage may be influenced, in part, by the acquisition of past tense regular verbs. That is, the use of regular verbs in the past tense may draw a child's attention to markers that distinguish between third person present tense and past tense for some irregular verbs.

If one adheres strictly to the developmental model of language teaching, the present tense would be taught before the regular past tense except for the third person singular. Next the clinician would teach the present tense, third person singular. There is one alternative, and that is to teach the present tense, third person singular before teaching the regular past tense without demanding the [-s], such as *he eat, she eat, it eat*. This tactic can be quickly rejected because it involves direct teaching of ungrammatical forms.

Now we are ready to examine premise 3. We first consider its implications for the processes of comprehension and production.

COMPREHENSION AND PRODUCTION

Language learning is still somewhat a mystery to psycholinguists. Some factors have been identified, and additionally some interesting hypotheses of the language learning process have been generated. It is now clear that children do not acquire language by accumulating stages of language achievement, as one would pile block upon block. Rather, children are exposed to a wide range of language input from which they sort out various bits and pieces, such that the end result gives the appearance of discrete developmental stages of achievement. Furthermore, the order in which language units are acquired reflects an overall progression of learning. It indicates neither the learning sequence nor the hypotheses about language that a child has entertained at each stage in development. In short, the developmental sequence indicates only *accomplishments*, not processes of language learning. Language acquisition is usually gauged by achievement in production. Perhaps for this reason language expression is often stressed in clinical practice. In contrast, parents do not teach language production. They are pleased, of course, when their children talk and even more pleased when the language shows a degree of maturity that makes conversation interesting. However, throughout the language learning process, parents do not directly *force* their children to produce language. They do, of course, encourage them to talk.

The term "forced production" needs explanation. Forced talking or forced production is defined here as a method of instruction that *requires* verbal responses from a child. Language clinicians try to force production from children in a number of ways.

One approach that is used to elicit verbal production is to have children acquire through imitation a word or sentence and then require that these memorized verbal utterances be used in response to a clinician's question or request to label objects or describe events. Sometimes clinicians ask a lot of questions and supply the appropriate answers. At other times clinicians paraphrase a child's response and ask him or her to repeat the paraphrase. All these approaches are artificial attempts to force a child to produce verbal responses. They are employed because it is believed that verbal production is essential to language learning.

The author would like to discourage the use of forced drills because he does not believe that language can be effectively taught in this manner. The evidence for this position is largely derived from knowledge of normal language development, which indicates that both meaningfulness and comprehensibility are important components of language development. But forced production is not necessarily part of this process. Parents create communicative experiences for their children. They motivate them to talk, they do not engage them in drills.

One of the dangers in using forced speaking drills is that it puts the individual into a handicapping situation. Have you ever been in a foreign language class where the teacher expected you to repeat long sentences or to answer questions when you were hardly able to understand the language? This is the position we place children in when we ask them to perform verbally before they fully understand what they are to say.

As far as can be determined, normally developing children are not specially trained to speak. Rather, their speaking reflects their underlying understanding about language and their willingness to communicate. McNeill (p. 69, 1966) illustrates this point with the following short excerpt.

Child: Nobody don't like me.
Mother: No, say "nobody likes me."
Child: Nobody don't like me.

After eight repetitions of this dialogue, the exasperated mother tried once more to correct her child's errors, saying, "No, now listen carefully; say '*nobody likes me.*'" To which the child responded, "Oh! Nobody don't likes me."

So it seems that children will not change until they understand the reason for changing. Correction can draw a person's attention to an error, but it is unlikely to do much more because correction alone does not provide sufficient and varied input to enable discovery of the relationships among the many parts of a language system.

Recent emphasis on pragmatics—the study of language functions (Searle, 1975)—has encouraged many clinicians to conclude that communication is the basic component through which language should be taught. If one were to contrast the difference between language training practices before 1975 and in the years following, it would seem that the emphasis now is largely on teaching language through communication. Syntactic or semantic structures are not ignored when communicative training is emphasized. They are taught indirectly in association with communicative functions (McLean and Snyder-McLean, 1978). In the past, some clinicians have advocated the communicative approach as the most reasonable and natural way to conduct language training. In this regard, the communicative (or pragmatic) approach is not a new concept in language teaching. In general, this teaching approach focuses on the use of language in communication. Through interesting games and activities, the young child is actively and thoroughly engaged in language training experiences. He or she hears language and often tries to respond with language.

Sometimes language exercises in the form of memorized dialogues, imitation drills, questions, and sentence construction drills are also used in combination with pragmatic experiences, but these exercises are not regarded as communicative activities, and, as we have discussed, probably do not facilitate language learning.

When using the communicative approach, the clinician will have certain linguistic objectives, such as emphasizing pronouns or prepositions, and will be guided by his or her understanding of normal language development. Additionally, the clinician will often talk in short uncomplicated sentences and repeat often. In most respects the conversation will be genuine because the activities are genuine.

Whenever possible, a second adult or normal speaking child should be a part of these activities. In this way the language delayed child can hear meaningful dialogue between two people. Drafting normal speaking children to participate in the games and activities is especially beneficial to the language delayed child because he or she can hear language that is communicative and age and task appropriate.

Each communicative centered task should have a *goal*. If, for example, a game is played in which a ball is to be rolled, a goal for this activity should be established that relates to the language structures that are to be emphasized. One such goal might be to roll the ball between two boxes, and to emphasize words such as near, far, between, and beyond. In this way the clinician can talk meaningfully to the child about "rolling the ball between the boxes." When the child misses, the clinician might spontaneously say, "You rolled the ball near the boxes. Now roll it between the boxes. Try again." A second activity is hand tracing. The clinician tells the children to trace their hands with crayon. When this activity has been completed, the clinician places the tracings on the floor and asks each child to find his or her own tracing by matching hand to tracing. In particular, the pronouns his/her/your/yours/mine can be emphasized. A third activity can involve the sorting of rocks. The clinician provides the children with a large box filled with different sizes of rocks. Each child is to take the rocks out and to help the clinician place the rocks in a line from large to small. Here adjectives of size are emphasized. Additionally, adjectival degree can be taught by introducing the words smaller, smallest, larger, and largest. The clinician does not force the children to talk in any of these activities, but provides experiences that encourage them to use language.

Communicative centered activities can include, for example, cleaning, grooming, or painting, but in all cases the activity should be *goal directed*. Each goal directed activity is designed to teach one or several language elements. When there is a goal, the language is meaningfully used, because both the clinician and the child are trying to complete an activity or accomplish a task, just as a parent and a child try to do in the environment of the home.

Forced production is not used when language is taught through the method of goal directed activities. Speaking is, of course, encouraged, but only indirectly. Throughout training, comprehension of language, through participation in meaningful communicative activities, takes priority. In this regard the primary role of the language clinician is: (1) to establish the structure, content, and function of language that is to be taught, using developmental norms as a guide, (2) to develop an appropriate communicative activity, and (3) to use language that is appropriate for the child, taking into account the child's language level and, if possible, his or her social and intellectual maturity. Through the use of goal directed communicative activity, interesting and functionally appropriate language will be used by the clinician and the child in a most natural way.

This approach that we have described has been used for some time to teach foreign languages (Asher, 1977; Winitz, 1981b). It is not a widely known method, but when used it has proved to be successful. Imagine having the opportunity to learn a foreign language without memorizing grammar—simply by engaging in communicative activities and listening. You would find it an enjoyable and highly profitable experience (Asher, 1977; Winitz, 1981b. A tape demonstrating comprehension training in Mandarin Chinese is available from International Linguistics Corp., 401 West 89th Street, Kansas City, Mo 64114. Films demonstrating this approach with second language learners are available from Sky Oaks Productions, 19544 Sky Oaks Way, Los Gatos, Calif. 95030.)

DEVELOPMENT OF EXPRESSIVE LANGUAGE

A question that is almost always asked is, How does speaking develop when the language training emphasizes only comprehension? Another question, almost as frequent, is, Should communicative oriented comprehension training be used when a child speaks fairly well, but makes only a few errors?

The first question is linked to the issue of the relation between comprehension and production. There are indications that for children learning their first language, and for adults acquiring a second language, speech will develop spontaneously when there has been sufficient comprehensible input (Winitz, 1981b). Even when normally intelligent individuals cannot speak because the speech mechanism is unable to operate properly, language apparently develops normally (Lenneberg, 1962; MacNeilage, Rootes, and Chase, 1967). However, these findings do not necessarily indicate that children who are delayed in language yet show some comprehension of language eventually will produce what they comprehend. There are studies that suggest this conclusion to be a strong possibility (Winitz, 1981c), but further research with language delayed children is necessary.

Even though there are children whose expressive abilities are severely limited, rarely is there a child who does not utter a few words. For example, 4-year-old children who speak in two-word phrases provide evidence that they can talk, but there are constraints that apparently prevent the production of sentences of greater length. Still there is not sufficient evidence from research on language delayed children that comprehension training alone will effect improvement. On the other hand, there is no evidence that comprehension training will *not* improve the language production skills of children.

Neither is there evidence that *language production exercises* will teach children to produce language. There have been clinical studies purporting to show this effect; but in these studies (e.g., Crystal et al., 1976), the children were involved in communicative activities and comprehension training, in addition to production practice.

There is, of course, the possibility that some children with language disorders comprehend language but are unable to convert this knowledge into production (Miller, 1981). However, there is no evidence to support this contention. Language delayed children are like normal children in that they often comprehend more than they can say, despite their lagging development of both comprehension and production. In the clinical treatment of language delayed children, there is the temptation, then, to consider children whose comprehension is in advance of their production to have a "disorder of language production." The next reasonable step, so it seems, is to begin production practice, to make the level of language production commensurate with the child's level of language comprehension. Again, there is no evidence that standard production training practices alone will result in an increased development of language production.

When production lags comprehension by a large amount, the primary teaching strategy still remains that of using communicative activities to motivate the child to talk. In this regard, comprehension is the primary channel through which language is received and through which additional language is learned.

Comprehension training does not always produce immediate dividends. That is, production does not result immediately from comprehension training through communication. There is sometimes a considerable lag in the development of these two skills (Winitz, 1981b). Patience is necessary because the effect of comprehension may not be realized for several months. Yet what is our alternative? Is it to try to force speech by asking a child to repeat a clinician's paraphrase or to engage in imitation drills, as implied in the discussion of premise 2. According to premise 2, training at the next higher level is to begin when all language elements for a developmental language level have been acquired. Premise 2 does not state when training at the next higher level should begin. It may be that moving to the next level almost immediately does not take into consideration the possibility that before production training is to begin at the next higher level a period should be devoted to production experience at the completed level.

We return now to the question of how to teach grammatical structures to children whose language is highly developed, but who show a few errors. For example, one frequent language error of children is the omission of the verb "to be" in certain contexts. Perhaps the most reasonable approach is to give children the opportunity to hear the standard speech forms in communicative contexts and to indicate to them that their patterns differ from the standard forms. That is, children should be made aware of the correct form. At no time should they be asked to distinguish between a correct form and an incorrect form, because hearing an incorrect form tends to establish it in the mind. They might be told to listen attentively or to identify the correct forms in passages. This approach is different from correcting a child's incorrect use of a form immediately after it has been uttered. Children who use nonstandard forms do not readily accept criticism largely because they don't understand the purpose or the reason for the correction. You can place yourself in the same situation. Suppose someone pointed out to you that you had incorrectly used *who* for *whom*. Would you learn this form? You might if *whom* were used correctly in standard conversational English, but of course, it is not; therefore, politely telling people to "mind" their who's and whom's is probably an ineffective teaching strategy.

In summary, teaching comprehension of language is a training methodology that emphasizes communication experiences through listening. In this approach, the developmental norms are used only as a framework to guide instruction. According to this approach, children are to *experience through listening* functionally relevant language, and they are to be placed in circumstances that motivate them to use expressive language. This approach to teaching language is in sharp contrast to current methods, which view language learning as the linear accumulation of developmental stages through practice in language production drills.

REFERENCES

Asher, J. 1977. Learning Another Language Through Actions, The Complete Teacher's Guidebook. Sky Oaks Productions, Los Gatos, Calif.

Bloom, L. 1970. Language Development: Form and Function in Emerging Grammars. MIT Press, Cambridge, Mass.

Bowerman, M. 1978a. Systematizing semantic knowledge: Changes over time in the child's organization of word meaning. Child Dev. 49:977–987.

Bowerman, M. 1978b. Words and sentences: Uniformity, individual variation, and shifts over time in patterns of acquisition. In: F. D. Minifie and L. L. Lloyd (eds.), Communicative and Cognitive Abilities—Early Behavioral Assessment. University Park Press, Baltimore.

Brown, R. 1973. A First Language, The Early Stages. Harvard University Press, Cambridge, Mass.

Butterworth, G., and Hatch, E. 1978. A Spanish-speaking adolescent's acquisition of English syntax. In: E. M. Hatch (ed.), Second Language Acquisition, A Book of Readings, Newbury House, Rowley, Mass.

Chapman, R. S. 1978. Comprehension strategies in children. In: J. F. Kavanagh and W. Strange (eds.), Speech and Language in the Laboratory, School, and Clinic. MIT Press, Cambridge, Mass.

Crystal, D., Fletcher, P., and Garman, M. 1976. The Grammatical Analysis of Language Disability. Edward Arnold, London.

Holland, A. L. 1975. Language therapy for children: Some thoughts on context and content. J. Speech Hear. Disord. 40:514–523.

Lahey, M., and Bloom, L. 1977. Planning a first lexicon: Which words to teach first. J. Speech Hear. Disord. 42:340–350.

Lenneberg, E. H. 1962. Understanding language without ability to speak: A case report. J. Abnorm. Social Psychol. 65:419–425.

McLean, J. E., and Snyder-McLean, L. K. 1978. A Transactional Approach to Early Language Training. Merrill, Columbus, Ohio.

MacNeilage, P. F., Rootes, T. P., and Chase, R. A. 1967. Speech production and perception in a patient with severe impairment of somesthetic perception and motor control. J. Speech Hear. Res. 10:449–467.

McNeill, D. 1966. Developmental psycholinguistics. In: F. Smith and G. A. Miller (eds.), The Genesis of Language, A Psycholinguistic Approach. MIT Press, Cambridge, Mass.

Miller, J. 1981. Assessing Language Production in Children: Experimental Procedures, Vol. I. University Park Press, Baltimore.

Miller, J. F., and Yoder, D. F. 1974. An ontogenetic language teaching strategy for retarded children. In: R. L. Schiefelbusch and L. L. Lloyd (eds.), Language Perspectives—Acquisition, Retardation, and Intervention. University Park Press, Baltimore.

Prutting, C. A. 1979. Process: The action of moving forward progressively from one point to another on the way to completion. J. Speech Hear. Disord. 44:3–30.

Searle, J. R. 1975. Speech acts and recent linguistics. In. D. Aaronson and R. W. Rieber (eds.), Developmental Psycholinguistics and Communication Disorders. Ann. New York Acad. Sci. Vol. 263.

Winitz, H. 1981a. Nonlinear learning and language teaching. In. H. Winitz (ed.), The Comprehension Approach to Foreign Language Instruction. Newbury House, Rowley, Mass.

Winitz, H. (ed.). 1981b. The Comprehension Approach to Foreign Language Instruction. Newbury House, Rowley, Mass.

Winitz, H. 1981c. A reconsideration of comprehension and production in language training. In: H. Winitz (ed.), The Comprehension Approach to Foreign Language Instruction. Newbury House, Rowley, Mass.

CHAPTER 4

Facilitating Comprehension, Recall, and Production of Language

Elaine Z. Lasky

Lasky's chapter emphasizes that language intervention procedures should capture the significant role that language plays in thought and communication. She challenges some traditional treatment approaches and proposes some new tactics for the language clinician.

1. *What is meant by levels of processing, and how does this concept relate to language teaching? How can this concept be implemented in language teaching?*
2. *What is a language learning strategy? How is it taught and what is its value?*
3. *Lasky suggests that language instruction should encompass the teaching of complex concepts? Identify the procedures that can be used to teach complex concepts.*
4. *Lasky speaks of adjusting the "evaluation procedure." What does this term mean, and how is the process carried out? Would you recommend it in all cases?*
5. *What are the goals of language intervention according to Lasky? How do these goals differ from your own goals?*

IN A TEACHING-LEARNING ENVIRONMENT, language is the vehicle for the presentation of old and new information, and frequently complex information. It is the vehicle through which children must often demonstrate their learning. Children with language disorders and learning disabilities, however, experience difficulties in comprehending language in the nursery or school classroom, language in school workbooks and texts, and language used by their classmates. They have difficulty remembering and assimilating language presented by their teachers and tutors. They have difficulty in using language for effective communication.

Speech-language pathologists can provide help for children with language disorders and learning disabilities if they acknowledge the complexity of the language children are expected to comprehend and use in the classroom, home, and playground, and do not ignore the social demands made on children outside the clinic. This chapter considers intervention procedures that take into account levels of language complexity with reference to the conceptual demands placed on children in the classroom, home, and social setting.

CURRENT ISSUES WITH DIRECT RELEVANCE FOR INTERVENTION

Activity and Intentions

We have become increasingly aware of the active involvement and participation with the environment that is normally sought by the child. We no longer describe the child as a passive observer. We see that activity is important for learning, and the greater the degree of active involvement with a task, at any age, the greater the learning (Brown, 1979; Nuttin, 1976). Even newborns interact with their environment, modifying their behavior to affect auditory experiences (Eilers and Oller, 1983; Trehub, Bull, and Schneider, 1981). Summarizing intensive work with infants under 6 months of age, Siqueland (1969) found no indication that the infant is a passive receiver of information; rather, the infant appears to seek out stimuli and activity. Soviet theories of activity reviewed by Brown (1979) emphasize the need in young children, as well as older children, for goal directed, involved, and meaningful activities for learning. Activity is directed by the child's intentions, motivational state, and interests (Weiner, 1976). Tasks that are tied to real-life interest produce greater effort and greater comprehension; intent to learn produces greater learning (Nuttin, 1976).

As clinicians, we need to program evaluation and treatment to keep the child actively involved with tasks that are challenging, meaningful, and goal directed. To sustain this attitude, we must examine critically treatment that makes extensive use of repetitious drills, requires simplistic or obvious responses, and encourages the child to remain somewhat passive and quiescent. Evaluation and treatment procedures, as discussed below, need to involve deep levels of processing and activity by the child.

Levels of Processing

In the levels of processing model, the depth of processing determines how elaborate and durable cognition and memory will be. A stimulus processed at a shallow level is transient and easily lost, whereas a trace processed more deeply to include meaning is more persistent and durable (Moates and Schumacher, 1980). The complexity of the required response, therefore, is seen to affect the level at which the information in the stimulus is processed; the level of processing, in turn, affects the comprehension and remembering of the stimulus (Craik and Tulving, 1975; Jacoby and Craik, 1979; Kintsch, 1979).

If a response requires interpreting the meaning of a stimulus, the stimulus will be processed at a deeper level, comprehended at a deeper level, and retained in memory for a longer period (Craik and Tulving, 1975; Jacoby and Craik, 1979; Kintsch, 1979). The progression is from shallow levels, such as indicating whether a word or phrase is in capital letters or contains a particular phoneme, to the number of syllables in a word, to imitating or repeating a word or sentence. Successively deeper levels are required to determine the syntactic category or to categorize the meaning of a word. Requiring a paraphrase or interpretation of a sentence requires still deeper processing; generating sentences that can logically follow the stimulus is even more involved.

Structuring learning tasks to help children process semantic, syntactic, and pragmatic aspects of language deeply enhances comprehension, learning, and memory. Requiring paraphrasing rather than imitation facilitates children's learning and remembering of a concept or construction. Requiring children to explain a principle or a linguistic rule involves still deeper processing and facilitates memory even more. To help promote active listening and recall, procedures can be planned so that the child in the clinic listens and states the missing last word of a _____ (Anderson, Goldberg, and Hidde, 1971; Kane and Anderson, 1977). The clinician presents a sentence; the child listens and supplies the necessary _____ . Practice in doing this overtly and then covertly (silently) in the clinic is followed by having the child attempt to do so in the classroom. This helps the child listen actively and process information more deeply. Kane and Anderson (1977) recommend structuring material to minimize the possibility of errors and yet to give practice in active listening with deeper processing. Other activities that involve deeper processing are role playing, explaining, and providing personal examples.

Use of Learning Strategies

What learning strategies do children need to know? Are they acquired without help? Children need to learn to attend and remember what the teacher says. Children need to learn what to listen to and how to listen (Cook-Gumperz, 1975), how to ask questions, and how to answer them (Norman and Bobrow, 1976). They need to develop techniques to organize information, and to acquire mnemonic strategies to store information in memory and to retrieve it from memory (Brown, 1977). They need to learn to evaluate the demands of the task and to understand their ability to meet these demands (Flavell and Wellman, 1977).

Most children develop these skills spontaneously from about the second or third grade and learn to refine them over the years to ages 11 or 12 (Brown, 1975; Brown, 1979; Naus and Halasz, 1979). Some children, however, do not acquire the necessary strategies for organizing, learning, and remembering (Bransford et al., 1980). Some exhibit difficulty in listening and picking out relevant information, asking a question, and evaluating what is needed for the task (Brown, 1979; Brown and Campione, 1978; Flavell and Wellman, 1977; Naus and Halasz, 1979). Many children with learning disabilities do not develop these strategies and proceed in an unplanned and unorganized manner (Schworm and Abelseth, 1981). They have difficulty in comprehending material, in selecting key ideas, in verbal reasoning, in determining cause and effect, and in making inferences (Kavale, 1980). They do not ask questions or verbalize meanings and interpretations as frequently as do children with normal learning skills (Wong, 1979).

We need to be aware of what strategies children use to enhance learning—to learn how to learn. We need to evaluate their use of strategies and to determine which may be relevant and helpful to children with language disorders. We need to help them develop these strategies.

PROCEDURES FOR EVALUATION
OF COMPREHENSION AND PRODUCTION OF LANGUAGE

Frequently Recommended Approaches

The facets of language to be assessed include phonology, syntax, semantics, and pragmatics. Comprehension and production of each must also be assessed. Among the most frequently used measures of comprehension of syntax and semantics are those that require picture pointing responses (Boehm, 1971; Carrow, 1973; Dunn, 1965). Imitation is a frequently used measure of language production (Carrow, 1974; Stephens, 1977; Zachman et al., 1978). Together these procedures may be used to sample syntactic constructions and semantic concepts that appear infrequently in a child's spontaneous speech, although it should be recognized that they reflect language performance under a restricted set of conditions.

With regard to the testing of comprehension, the exclusive use of recognition and picture pointing tasks may provide information that is not entirely correct because children sometimes respond to cues other than the focal linguistic unit (Shipley, 1980). Errors in performance may be due to many factors: ambiguity (Haynes and McCallion, 1981) or an inappropriate level of abstraction of the items (Washington and Naremore, 1978; Woznak and Lasky, 1980), attractiveness or salience of alternative items (Rizzo and Stephens, 1981), contradictions that result from a child's background or certain personal expectations (Nelson, 1979; Strohner and Nelson, 1974), bias caused by greater familiarity with certain items (Bransford and Nitsch, 1978; Chapandy and Lasky, 1980), or the way task instructions are given (Bahrick, 1979; Jacoby and Craik, 1979).

Similarly the value of using elicited imitation to assess language production is problematic. There is some evidence that utterances can be imitated without being processed fully (Fraser, Bellugi, and Brown, 1963; Lovell and Dixon, 1965; Miller, 1981), and, therefore, sometimes can reflect incorrectly linguistic competence (Hood and Lightbown, 1978; Miller and Yoder, 1973). Under normal circumstances, individuals do not store and repeat sentences verbatim, but put the gist of the meaning in memory. What is stored is related to the context of the situation and what is known about the topic or event. Therefore, a child who fails to imitate correctly may be reflecting a personal interpretation of the test utterance, and may not have a disorder in language competence or auditory memory (Norman, 1976). Although helpful in some instances, elicited imitation should be a supplemental procedure.

Consider Language Level and Task Difficulty I challenge the emphasis or exclusive use of picture pointing, elicited imitation, and similar formats to evaluate language comprehension and production. The rationale for the challenge: picture pointing is rarely an adequate response for a school age child in a social setting, home environment, or classroom. Also, imitation, as a frequent or typical response, is not effective for any child above 2 years of age in any situation. Speech-language clinicians must evaluate a child's communicative competence. To make this evaluation, we need to examine the types of stimulus presented to children in the classroom, on the playground, and in the home, and the types of response that are required.

Tasks that require solving problems, making judgments, drawing conclusions, and using social perceptual skills go beyond the level of task difficulty required of most language tests. However, the tests children take in the classroom contain questions that use these higher skills. Even in the primary grades, the information presented and the response tasks that are required often demand comprehension and production of complex concepts embedded in complex and/or conjoined sentences in paragraphs. In one readiness test designed for beginning to middle kindergarten, the children are required to select a picture from one of four similar pictures, by making inferences from complex statements, for example, "Mrs. Green got her camera, put some film in it, and took her baby outside. Mark what Mrs. Green wanted to make." (Nurss and McGauvran, 1976). In workbooks used in the first grade, children are to recall details, and to sequence, interpret, and make inferences from a story they have read. They need to answer such questions as "What is a riddle?" or explain such statements as "It's a dog's life." (Schaubert, Goldberg, and Lane, 1976). They need to supply appropriate morphemes for tenses, plurals, comparatives, and adverbs, to make contractions, and to put items in alphabetical order (Richardson, Smith, and Weiss, 1965). Third grade science texts contain statements such as "A habitat factor is any part of a habitat with which a population can interact." Children then must find habitat factors for mice and answer the question, "How do mice interact with each factor?" (Berger et al., 1974).

In the higher grades, the concepts become more difficult as does the level of responding. Ninth to twelfth grade students are, for example, shown a graph and statistics regarding the gross national product and asked to consider the impact on GNP of rising costs of cleaning polluted lakes and streams. They are told to ". . . decide whether or not the change in figures would represent any real change in the economic well being of Americans." (Judd, 1975). These examples illustrate the complexity of language constructions and levels of thinking and decision making that are required in the typical classroom setting. Can we evaluate adequately children with language disorders with tasks that require lower level responses?

Consider the Testing Environment   Traditional language testing is administered in the language clinic, where conditions are generally more favorable for using language than in the classroom (Lasky, 1983). Let us look briefly at the clinic in which evaluation and treatment take place. In this one-on-one or small group clinical setting, the relevant signal or stimulus is generally presented in quiet, without distractions or message competitors; one speaker talks at a time. In responding to a question or taking a turn, the child may act without delay, whenever he or she chooses. Evaluation is done individually or in small groups of other children who may also have speech and language disorders. The clinician is not only sympathetic but involved with this small group.

Work in the classroom, however, necessitates listening, responding, doing seat work, and taking tests in a large group setting. Several factors may affect performance. First, competing auditory stimuli from other persons who are speaking are likely to disrupt or distract a child's attention to a teacher's presentation (Lasky and Tobin, 1973). Second, in the classroom, children can rarely respond immediately to questions from the teacher. They must wait to be called on before responding. They must learn to wait until all instructions have been given and all their classmates' questions have been answered before proceeding. Waiting, then, creates a delay and requires use of memory before answering. Third, the presence of other students or other observers in the classroom may create for the child social stress, which may interfere in various ways with comprehension and production of language. Fourth, factors such as rate of speech, stress patterns, structural complexity, and redundancy may contribute to a child's difficulty in the comprehension and production of language. The rate of presentation by the clinician may be considerably slower than that of the classroom teacher. Additionally, the teacher's speech may contain different stress patterns and be structurally more complex and less redundant.

Adjusting Evaluation Procedures

When we recognize that language in the classroom is complex, that language involves several levels of responding, and that competing messages and delayed responses must be considered (Lasky, 1983), how should we go about the assessment of language?

We should evaluate comprehension and production with materials that represent the semantic, syntactic, and pragmatic complexity of the classroom. We should be flexible. Not all procedures are for every child, nor every procedure for any child. We should evaluate the child's semantic level with concepts used in the classroom. At the lower grade levels, items from the Test of Basic Concepts (Boehm, 1971) can be used to assess the comprehension of concepts. Since this test is a picture pointing test, the clinician should follow up by selecting a few items from the test for evaluation of higher levels of responding. For example, the clinician can ask the child to explain an item, to use an item in a sentence, or to create a story from an item. Additional test items can be selected from curriculum materials used in the child's class.

The clinician may check comprehension of concepts by testing them in simple sentences, then in sentences of increasing syntactic complexity. For example, does the child comprehend the concept when it is used in an embedded sentence as part of the main clause, as a relative clause, or as a complement? Also, does the child use the concept with logical conjunctions, such as *and, or, nor, if-then, except, but, until, before-after, although*? Have the child explain and respond to Wh-questions and Wh-pronouns. Does the child know when and how to ask a question? Does the child recognize and interpret idiomatic expressions (You're pulling my leg), riddles, puns, and jokes?

Few tests routinely assess these more complex and difficult activities. The subtests of several tests can be used to elicit some of this information (Baker and Leland, 1967; Newcomer and Hammill, 1977; Semel and Wiig, 1980). However, in most cases the language clinician must improvise.

Alter Environment to Simulate Classroom   To evaluate performance under conditions that reflect the classroom environment, a clinician may use a tape recorder to simulate the competing auditory messages of the classroom. Do the competing auditory messages affect comprehension or production of language? To what messages do the children attend? Are they easily distracted under this condition?

Evaluate performance when the child's response is delayed. Have the child hold an answer to a question for 5 to 10 seconds to simulate the classroom. Does performance change? How? Does performance change in terms of number correct and/or adequacy of completeness?

Present sentences or instructions at a normal rate, about 150 words per minute (WPM). Slow the rate to 120 WPM. Is comprehension affected? Is behavior altered? Observe the children in the classroom during a listening and learning period, as well as when they do seat work or take a test. How does each child comprehend and produce language in a classroom setting? A set of specific questions can also be given to the classroom teacher or special teacher to obtain information about performance in the classroom.

Gather Data on Communicative Competence in Social Settings   Question the teacher and the family to gather information on behavior in different forms of social interaction. Does the child communicate at home? Does the child relate to the parent any information about items studied in school or events that occurred on the playground? Are there daily communication exchanges at home? How does the child explain needs and wants at home?

How does the child communicate with peers in social groups at school or in the neighborhood? I frequently ask clinicians about their concern with a child who is doing poorly academically but well socially, as opposed to a child who does well academically but poorly socially. Invariably, they report more concern about the child who is at a social disadvantage. Most suggest, however, that they rarely evaluate or work to improve social communication. We should include observation and evaluation of children with language disorders in social communication settings.

The evaluation format discussed above emphasizes the assessment of comprehension and production of language that reflects the level of difficulty of the classroom and social environments. The evaluation procedures should include testing under quiet, and under competing auditory messages, and should provide the comparing of delayed and immediate responses for slow and normal rates of presentation. These evaluation procedures spell out a rather straightforward and workable intervention.

Intervention

Select Semantic Concepts and Syntactic Constructions   Begin by selecting semantic concepts needed for communicating and learning in the classroom. Which concepts were comprehended during the evaluation? Which presented problems? Teach simpler semantic concepts, then build to the more difficult concepts that are relevant and necessary for the classroom.

Teach concepts in isolation, in short phrases, in simple sentences, and then in constructions of increasing syntactic complexity, such as embedded sentences and sentences using logical conjunctions. Present new concepts with easier or lower level tasks, such as recognition, picture pointing, or modeling. Gradually increase the level of complexity. At first use cued recall. Later use recall without cueing, as the concept is reviewed and the child gains greater comprehension. Use contextual cues and dramatic explanations to help the child integrate the concept and later retrieve it from memory. Try to elaborate the memory trace to help to facilitate retrieval. Use concrete examples with names of children and teachers he or she knows. Use imagery with absurd or funny examples. Ask the child to tell why it is funny. Increase the level of response difficulty by teaching paraphrasing, by explaining, and by using concepts to teach children how to make inferences and draw conclusions.

Increase Difficuty of Presentation, Task, and Materials   At first present the concept in the clinic at a slower than normal rate of 120 WPM, then increase the rate to an average, normal rate, about 150 to 180 WPM. Present the semantic-syntactic stimuli in quiet as new information is taught. With review or with easier work, gradually add competing talkers, either simulated via tape recorder, or with other children talking in the clinic room. Use the competing auditory messages with a favorable signal-to-noise (S/N) ratio first. Again, while reviewing, gradually increase the level of the competing messages to a less favorable but realistic S/N ratio, such as +10 dB. Give the children opportunities to work on varieties of tasks under varying levels of competing talkers. Allow them to work individually with you, in small groups, or with paper and pencil or crayon tasks that simulate classroom seat work. Help them to learn to monitor or check their concentration under conditions of competing messages.

When presenting new or complex information, allow children to respond as soon as they wish. When reviewing or presenting simpler information, have the children delay responses rather than answer immediately. If the children have difficulty doing this, teach them to acquire strategies to facilitate remembering, such as rehearsing or chunking (combining) units.

The clinician can use different activities to provide practice, yet each should challenge the child to become an active participant. Many of the materials developed for clinicians seem to be appropriate for the very young child, the nursery aged, or kindergarten aged child, but challenging materials are needed for the older child (Wiig and Semel, 1980). A wide variety of activities can be adapted by clinicians from language arts materials. Numerous paperback books are available in bookstores and libraries to help with idioms, riddles, and jokes. Two- or three-line jokes can be useful to get at dual meanings in language. Workbooks are available at primary through high school grade levels to help a child acquire skills for drawing conclusions, following directions, getting the main idea, and using context (Boning, 1979).

Include Social Learning When Teaching Communicative Competence Role playing, verbalizing about feelings, and problem solving are valuable techniques for teaching social sensitivity and interpersonal skills. The "What would you do if..." format is useful, as are the "How do you think he..." and "What should she do if ..." approaches. For example, my students located a workbook designed to help develop social awareness through the use of short vignettes. Topics included asking for an explanation of a child's worries, discussing a child's negative behaviors, talking about a child's interpretation of a situation, and considering how to pick a pal (Fornette, Forte, and Harris, 1979).

Clinician Acts as Indirect Service Component We think of the clinician as providing direct service to children. To increase our efficiency and to facilitate the children's progress, we need to build several support systems. We should serve as consultants to help teachers and specialists work directly with the children. We should work with parents and/or siblings. We should train and meticulously monitor peer tutors. For these support efforts to work, we need to keep the clients apprised of our work and we need to learn their feelings about their work at home, in the classroom, and with the tutor.

This chapter has considered the preparation a language disordered child needs to function adequately in the classroom and in social settings. The training should involve deep levels of language processing and should closely approximate the level of difficulty observed in the classroom. Suggestions for direct service by clinicians were presented, as were suggestions for including teachers, other specialists, parents, and peers.

REFERENCES

Anderson, R. C., Goldberg, S. R., and Hidde, J. L. 1971. Meaningful processing of sentences. J. Educ. Psychol. 62:395–399.

Bahrick, H. 1979. Broader methods and narrower theories for memory research: Comments on the papers by Eysenck and Cermak. In: L. Cermak and F. Craik (eds.), Levels of Processing in Human Memory, pp. 141–158. Lawrence Erlbaum Associates, Hillsdale, N.J.

Baker, H., and Leland, B. 1967. Detroit Test of Learning Aptitude. Test Division of Bobbs-Merrill, Indianapolis.

Berger, C. F., Berkheimer, G. D., Lewis, J. E. Jr., Neuberger, H. T., and Wood, E. A. 1974. Modular Activities Program in Science. Houghton-Mifflin, Boston.

Boehm, A. 1971. Boehm Test of Basic Concepts. Psychological Corporation, New York.

Boning, R. A. 1979. Specific Skill Series. Barnell Loft, Ltd., Baldwin, N.Y.

Bransford, J. D., and Nitsch, K. E. 1978. Coming to understand things we could not previously understand. In: J. F. Kavanagh and W. Strange (eds.), Speech and Language in the Laboratory, School, and Clinic, pp. 267–307. MIT Press, Cambridge, Mass.

Bransford, J., Stein, B., Shelton, T., and Owings, R. 1980. Cognition and adaptation: The importance of learning to learn. In: J. Harvey (ed.), Cognition, Social Behavior and the Environment, pp. 93–110. Lawrence Erlbaum Associates, Hillsdale, N.J.

Brown, A. L. 1975. The development of memory: Knowing, knowing about knowing, and knowing how to know. In: H. W. Reese (ed.), Advances in Child Development and Behavior, pp. 104–152, Vol. 10. Academic Press, New York.

Brown, A. L. 1977. Development, schooling, and the acquisition of knowledge about knowledge. In: R. C. Anderson, R. J. Spiro, and W. E. Montague (eds.), Schooling and the Acquisition of Knowledge, pp. 241–253. Lawrence Erlbaum Associates, Hillsdale, N.J.

Brown, A. L. 1979. Theories of memory and the problems of development: Activity, growth, and knowledge. In: L. Cermak and F. Craik (eds.), Levels of Processing in Human Memory, pp. 225–258. Larence Erlbaum Associates, Hillsdale, N.J.

Brown, A. L., and Campione, J. C. 1978. Memory strategies in learning: Training children to study strategically. In: H. L. Pick, Jr., H. W. Leibowitz, J.

E. Singer, A. Steinschneider, and H. W. Stevenson (eds.), Psychology: From Research to Practice, pp. 47–73. Plenum Press, New York.

Carrow, E. 1973. Test for Auditory Comprehension of Language. Learning Concepts, Austin, Tex.

Carrow, E. 1974. Carrow Elicited Language Inventory. Learning Concepts, Austin, Tex.

Chapandy, A., and Lasky, E. 1980. The effect of word familiarity on children's comprehension and memory. Ohio J. Speech Hear. 15:1–11.

Cook-Gumperz, J. 1975. The child as a practical reasoner. In: M. Sanches and B. G. Blount (eds.), Language Thought, and Culture, pp. 137–162. Academic Press, New York.

Craik, F. I. M., and Tulving, E. 1975. Depth of processing and the retention of words in episodic memory. J. Exp. Psychol. Gen. 104:268–294.

Dunn, L. M., 1965. Peabody Picture Vocabulary Test. American Guidance Service, Circle Pines, Minn.

Eilers, R. E., and Oller, D. K., 1983. Speech perception in infancy and early childhood. In: E. Lasky and J. Katz (eds.), Central Auditory Processing Disorders: Problems of Speech, Language, and Learning. University Park Press, Baltimore.

Flavell, J. H., and Wellman, H. M. 1977. Metamemory, In: R. V. Kail, Jr., and J. W. Hagen (eds.), Perspectives on the Development of Memory and Cognition. pp. 3–33. Lawrence Erlbaum Associates, Hillsdale, N.J.

Fornette, C., Forte, I., and Harris, B. 1979. A Social Awareness Activity Book. Incentive Publications, Nashville, Tenn.

Fraser, C., Bellugi, U., and Brown, R. 1963. Control of grammar in imitation and comprehension and production. J. Verb. Learn. Verb. Behav. 2:121–135.

Haynes, W. O., and McCallion, M. B. 1981. Language comprehension testing: The influence of three modes of test administration and cognitive tempo on the performance of preschool children. Lang. Speech Hear. Serv. Schools 12:74–81.

Hood, L., and Lightbown, P. 1978. What children do when asked to "Say what I say": Does elicited imitation measure linguistic knowledge? Allied Health Behav. Sci. 1:195–219.

Jacoby, L., and Craik, F. 1979. Effects of elaboration of processing and encoding and retrieval: Trace distinctiveness and recovery of initial context. In: L. Cermak and F. Craik (eds.), Levels of Processing in Human Memory, pp. 1–22. Lawrence Erlbaum Associates, Hillsdale, N.J.

Judd, B. 1975. Teacher's Guide for a New History of the United States: An Inquiry Approach. Holt, Rinehart and Winston, New York.

Kane, J. H., and Anderson, R. C. 1977. Depth of processing and interference efforts in the learning and remembering of sentences. Technical Report 21, Center for the Study of Reading. University of Illinois Press, Urbana.

Kavale, K. A. 1980. Learning disability and cultural economic disadvantage: The case for a relationship. Learn. Disability Q. 3:97–112.

Kintsch, W. 1979. Levels of processing language material: Discussion of the papers by Lachman and Lachman and Perfetti. In: L. Cermak and F. Craik (eds.), Levels of Processing in Human Memory, pp. 211–222. Lawrence Erlbaum Associates, Hillsdale, N.J.

Lasky, E. Z. 1983. An overview of the parameters affecting auditory processing. In: E. Lasky and J. Katz (eds.), Central Auditory Processing Disorders: Problems of Speech, Language, and Learning. University Park Press, Baltimore.

Lasky, E. Z., and Tobin, H. 1973. Linguistic and nonlinguistic competing message effects. J. Learn. Disabilities. 6:243–250.

Lovell, J., and Dixon, E. 1965. The growth of the control of grammar in imitation, comprehension and production. J. Child Psychol. Psychiatr. 14:123–138.

Miller, J. F. 1981. Assessing Language Production in Children: Experimental Procedures. Vol. I. University Park Press, Baltimore.

Miller, J. F., and Yoder, D. 1973. Assessing the comprehension of grammatical form in mentally retarded children. Paper presented at the International Association for the Scientific Study of Mental Deficiency, September 1973, The Hague, Netherlands. As cited in J. F. Miller, 1981. Assessing Language Production in Children: Experimental Procedures, p. 176. Vol. I. University Park Press, Baltimore.

Moates, D. R., and Schumacher, G. M. 1980. An Introduction to Cognitive Psychology. Wadsworth, Belmont, Calif.

Naus, M., and Halasz, F. 1979. Developmental perspectives on cognitive processing and semantic memory structure. In: L. Cermak and F. Craik (eds.), Levels of Processing in Human Memory, pp. 259–288. Lawrence Erlbaum Associates, Hillsdale, N.J.

Nelson, D. 1979. Remembering pictures and words: Appearance, significance, and name. In: L. Cermak and F. Craik (eds.), Levels of Processing in Human Memory, pp. 45–76. Lawrence Erlbaum Associates, Hillsdale, N.J.

Newcomer, P. L., and Hammill, D. D. 1977. The Test of Language Development. Empiric Press, Austin, Tex.

Norman, D. A. 1976. Memory and Attention, 2nd Ed. Wiley, New York.

Norman, D. A., and Bobrow, D. G. 1976. On the role of active memory processes in perception and cognition. In: C. N. Cofer (ed.), The Structure of Human Memory, pp. 114–132. Freeman, San Francisco.

Nurss, J. R., and McGauvran, M. E. 1976. Metropolitan Readiness Tests. Level 1, Form P. Harcourt Brace Jovanovich, New York.

Nuttin, J. R. 1976. Motivation and reward. In: W. K. Estes (ed.), Handbook of Learning and Cognitive Processes: Human Learning and Motivation, pp. 247–281. Vol. 3. Lawrence Erlbaum Associates, Hillsdale, New Jersey.

Richardson, J. E. Jr., Smith, H. L., Jr., and Weiss, B. J. 1965. Letters, Patterns, and Drills. The Linguistic Readers. Teacher's Ed. Harper Row, New York.

Rizzo, J. M., and Stephens, M. I. 1981. Performance of children with normal and impaired oral language production on a set of auditory comprehension tests. J. Speech Hear. Disord. 46:150–159.

Schaubert, E. D., Goldberg, E. S., and Lane, B. M. 1976. Socks and Secrets, Reading Basics Plus. Teacher's Ed. Harper Row, New York.

Schworm, R. W., and Abelseth, J. L. 1981. Evaluating instructional interactions: Where do we begin teaching? Learn. Disability Q. 4:101–111.

Semel, E. M., and Wiig, E. H. 1980. Clinical Evaluation of Language Functions (CELF). Charles E. Merrill, Columbus, Ohio.

Shipley, K. G. 1980. Interpreting results obtained from Carrow's TACL. J. Speech Hear. Disord. 46:222–223.

Siqueland, E. R. 1969. The development of instrumental exploratory behavior during the first year of human life. Paper presented at the Biennial Meeting of the Society for Research in Child Development, March, Santa Monica, Calif. As cited in B. Friedlander, G. Steritt, and G. Kirk (eds.), Exceptional Infant, Assessment and Intervention, pp. 84–109. Vol. 3. Bruner Mazel, New York.

Stephens, I. 1977. Stephens Oral Language Screening Test. Interim Publishers, Peninsula, Ohio.

Strohner, H., and Nelson, K. 1974. The young child's development of sentence comprehension: Influence of event probability, nonverbal context, syntactic form and strategies. Child Dev. 45:567–576.

Trehub, S. E., Bull, D., and Schneider, B. A. 1981. Infant speech and nonspeech perception: A review and reevaluation. In: R. L. Schiefelbusch and D. Bricker (eds.), Early Language: Acquisition and Intervention, pp. 9–50. University Park Press, Baltimore.

Washington, D. S., and Naremore, R. C. 1978. Children's use of spatial prepositions in two- and three- dimensional tasks. J. Speech Hear. Res. 21:151–165.

Weiner, B. 1976. Motivation from the cognitive perspective. In: W. K. Estes (ed.), Handbook of Learning and Cognitive Processes: Human Learning and Motivation, pp. 283–308. Vol. 3. Lawrence Erlbaum Associates, Hillsdale, N.J.

Wiig, E. H., and Semel, E. M. 1980. Language Assessment and Intervention for the Learning Disabled. Charles E. Merrill, Columbus, Ohio.

Wong, B. Y. L. 1979. Increasing retention of main ideas through questioning strategies. Learn. Disability Q. 2:42–47.

Woznak, D., and Lasky, E. Z. 1980. Levels of visual abstraction and the assessment of language comprehension in trainable mentally retarded children. J. Child. Commun. Disord. 4:12–18.

Zachman, L., Huisingh, R., Jorgesen, C., and Barrett, M. 1978. The Oral Language Sentence Imitation Screening Test/The Oral Language Sentence Imitation Diagnostic Inventory (OLSIST/OLSIDI) Statistical Manual. Lingui Systems, Moline, Ill.

CHAPTER 5

Curriculum Concepts for Language Treatment of Children

Lawrence J. Turton

Turton views language teaching as a comprehensive curriculum of instruction. He provides a detailed and principled basis for this approach, taking into account normal language development, individual differences, testing considerations, and procedures for treatment and evaluation.

1. *Turton uses the term "language curriculum." How does he define this term? What are its five characteristics?*
2. *Turton recommends that language instruction be based on normal language development. What are some of the reasons underlying this recommendation? Would you add any others?*
3. *What is "criterion referenced" evaluation in language assessment? How does this approach differ from "norm referenced" testing? What special knowledge must a clinician have to do criterion referenced evaluations? Can norms be used in criterion referenced testing? What are some practical ways to implement "criterion referenced" testing?*
4. *According to Turton, "attention" is fundamental in language acquisition. How does he use this term? How is the concept of "salient stimulus" used with regard to the process of attention?*
5. *How does Turton view the process of imitation in language learning? What does he mean by "matching" the responses of others? Do you agree?*
6. *Turton defines discrimination as a basic learning strategy. How does this strategy contribute to language learning?*

7. *How does Turton suggest that IEP goals be changed to take into account the various processes of language learning? Is this easy to do? In this regard, how does he distinguish between "the behavioral manipulation of language structures" and the "fostering of language acquisition"? Is there a real difference in actual practice? If so, what procedures would you identify with each approach?*

8. *What procedures are available for evaluating improvement in language? How does Turton differentiate a formal from an informal evaluation? Distinguish among continuous recordings, probes, and structural observations, three procedures proposed by Turton for evaluating language. On the basis of Turton's discussion of evaluation, what procedures would you favor?*

IN THE PAST TWO DECADES, language treatment for children has experienced a significant change in terms of its conceptual base and procedures for implementation. We have moved from a medical-diagnostic system to a developmental-psychoeducational model for treatment. We are moving from a treatment perspective of eliciting speech to one of facilitating communication and the acquisition of linguistic rules. Above all else, we are placing language once again into the cognitive-social sphere of human development.

Because speech-language pathology is an applied field, the knowledge base for this shift has come from the basic research fields of cognitive psychology, linguistics, behavioral psychology, and human development. Our contribution as a discipline has been the transformation of the basic research findings from theoretical-inductive statements to general principles of language treatment. There are a number of risks involved in this dependence on other professions, not the least of which is the problem of "appeal to authority"; that is, the manifestation of an attitude that because a finding appears in a journal or text, it should not be critically scrutinized. A clinician cannot wait for theorists to demonstrate the validity of a theory before translating the principles into a treatment program. Often, clinical judgment must be used to interpret, amplify, and extend research findings.

This chapter focuses on one aspect of the shift to the developmental-psychoeducational model, namely, the trend toward a developmentally sequenced program for facilitating language acquisition. In educational terms, the shift is from planning on a session-to-session basis to a predetermined sequence of teaching objectives, strategies, and evaluations, that is, a curriculum sequence. Individualized teaching no longer means attempting to isolate gaps or deficiencies in development; instead, it now means attempting to determine the child's level of language functioning and to expand on it. The task is not an easy one, nor is it as precise as one could want. But it does provide a system featuring direct relations between assessment and treatment, between objectives and strategies.

DEFINITION OF LANGUAGE CURRICULUM

Because the word "curriculum" has many connotations, an understanding of its application to language instruction must be predicated on a set of chracteristics that have a modicum of agreement in the professional literature. Consequently, this chapter is based on a theory of curriculum as an instructional manifestation of developmental principles. These principles have evolved primarily from the findings on normal development and instructional processes rather than classroom based teaching of academic subjects. Conceptually, however, there is one similarity; learning is viewed as a sequential, hierarchical process, with adequate performance outside the instructional setting being the ultimate criterion of success. Just as a student's ability to use reading as a functional tool in the real world is the final measure of reading instruction, the child's ability to communicate in his or her environment is the anticipated outcome of language instruction.

A language curriculum can best be defined as a process for teaching a child how to acquire the cognitive-perceptual bases of language and to manifest this knowledge in a set of linguistic rules. Language instruction is not a set of procedures to teach the child how to produce a restricted set of words or sentences. Instead, it is a process to teach the child how to acquire information from the environment, to organize this information into cognitive schemata, and to generate linguistic rules and forms from these schemata. The primary emphasis on language instruction must be on the principles and strategies of acquisition (i.e., how children learn to talk); the production of such specific language forms as words and sentences is secondary to the strategies and is an outcome of a correctly sequenced pattern of instruction.

There are five fundamental characteristics of language curriculum that can be abstracted from the literature:

1. Specification of the model of language acquisition
2. Specification of the target population
3. Specification of the strategies of instruction
4. Specification of the outcomes of instruction
5. Specification of the procedures for evaluation

A comprehensive curriculum for language acquisition should include these five characteristics as a minimum. Without adherence to these factors, language instruction will be reduced in its effectiveness and will result in a less than normal system for the child.

This chapter explores each of the five curriculum characteristics relative to its application in the design and implementation of language instruction. Throughout, the discussion emphasizes the relation between the normal processes of acquisition and procedures for teaching children. Essentially, we focus on the language clinician as a developmental specialist, a theme advanced in an earlier text (Turton, 1982). Indeed, language instruction can be viewed as an outcome of developmental intervention, not clinical intervention. The clinician is a child developmentalist who happens to be interested in communication processes. A viable curriculum guides the specialist through the process

of instruction, ensuring that the adult helps the child through all sequences. In many respects, it is written for the clinician as a format
for decision making rather than as a sequence of objectives for the
child.

SPECIFICATION OF MODEL OF LANGUAGE ACQUISITION

Language instruction must be based on normal language development—a self-evident but easily forgotten dictum. Language instruction, far too often, is equated with expanding phrase or sentence length
according to assumptions about syntactic rules. What is disregarded
is the totality of language performance, that is, its social-cognitive-
pragmatic prerequisites, as well as the grammatical form of the response. Often we start teaching by emphasizing the development of
vocabulary. Once we move to phrases, we slip into the trap of spoken
responses becoming the focal point of treatment. We repeatedly forget
that the goal is to teach the child how to produce a set of utterances,
not to emit an oral response to auditory, visual, or verbal stimuli.

A carefully planned, sequenced curriculum helps to prevent the
clinician from falling into the narrow objectives of the individualized
education program (IEP) requirement set forth in PL 94-142, the Education of All Handicapped Children Act. The clinician should start
by making a careful review of some of the common principles of acquisition.

1. Cognition is the ultimate controlling factor in the developmental
   process for language. It provides the child, *at all levels of development*, with the content of communication and the strategies for
   communication (Bloom and Lahey, 1978; Slobin, 1973).
2. Language is a social act that occurs in an environmental context.
   The context forms the pragmatic basis for communication.
   Through the social context, the child learns how and when to communicate; communication becomes one aspect of the interaction
   among humans (Bates, 1976).
3. The task for childhood is to learn to learn. The cognitive system
   includes at least two components: strategies of acquisition and the
   product of the strategies, the schemata of the world. Language
   instruction must focus on both so that the child can learn to abstract
   information from the environment as well as to produce utterances.
   Information about the structure of language is as important as the
   meaning of a word.
4. Language is frequently described as being comprised of five systems or levels: pragmatics, semantics, syntax, morphology, and

phonology. Language is also a function that involves comprehension and production of the five levels, predicated on the child's level of cognitive development. Instruction that focuses only on production is developmentally inappropriate.

5. Utterances can vary in meaning and function according to context. Words and sentences can have different meanings in different situations. Children need to learn the various meanings based on use and context. Careful attention must be given to teaching the depth of semantics as well as the breadth (Bloom and Lahey, 1978).

6. Language is sequential and hierarchical. One type of utterance is evolved from another. New information is learned from old. This concept applies not only to form and content as suggested by Slobin; it applies also to the interactions of the social-cognitive-linguistic systems. Development is not linear; it is geometrical and can only be taught from that perspective (Slobin, 1973).

7. Children do not start to speak with adult forms. Normal children follow a special "dialectical" model of development; handicapped children should be given the same opportunity. Evaluation must be predicated on normal child patterns, not viewed as correct or incorrect adult responses (Turton, 1982; Turton and Clark, 1971).

8. Social environments, especially play, form the learning contexts for normal children. Language instruction must always be put into this context. Play can be structured and goal oriented; natural consequences are powerful reinforcers. The traditional one-to-one treatment arrangement is appropriate for instruction for very specific forms and as a format for teaching the child how to respond. But the response must be placed in an environmental context as soon as possible (Liebergott, 1978).

All these principles can and should be used in the instructional process from the beginnings of the first words through the refinement of conversation. Before the clinician initiates the instructional process, the curriculum should be specified, detailed, and sequenced. It is only through the curriculum that the clinician can select the objectives, the teaching strategies, the environmental contexts, and the evaluation procedures. It is only through the curriculum that the clinician can demonstrate his or her knowledge of normal development.

After the passage of PL 94-142, there was inordinate emphasis on the IEP, to the detriment of curricular development for handicapped children. A premise of this chapter is that language instruction and other developmental-educational areas can only be strengthened by the publication of curricula derived from developmental principles. If one starts by acknowledging that human behavior has universal, common traits, then a language curriculum is an expression of the universalities of the developmental process for language. It is better to abstract specific goals for individuals (and IEPs) from these universal statements, than to view each child as having a unique set of language skills and problems.

SPECIFICATION OF TARGET POPULATION

Language instruction is a product of the interaction of three variables: the child, the clinician, and the cognitive-linguistic demands of the culture. The contribution of each variable changes with each clinical situation. Although each child is expected to leave treatment with a normal language system, the pacing of the acquisition of such a system will be a function of what the child brings to the instructional setting and how the clinician adapts to the status of the child.

From the medical-diagnostic orientation, the profession learned to stress differential diagnosis and assignment to a category as the basis for adapting treatment to the child. The childhood aphasic was viewed as being different from the hearing impaired or mentally retarded child. Treatment was "therapy" to overcome or remediate deficits.

Because of the influence of theories of behaviorism, we shifted from diagnostic categorization of children to the polar position that the child's related problems were irrelevant and that a clinician could teach any child any behavior or skill merely through the arrangement of stimuli and contingencies. Language content, thus, became the only significant variable and, within the concept of language, usually only syntactic responses and their length received emphasis. Lost in this conceptualization were the developmental differences among children, which are reflected in the diagnostic categories. The child became a passive participant in the equation for instruction.

Testing Models

Just as cognitive-linguistic theory has affected the model for language acquisition, it has also impacted on how we evaluate the status of the child and the pattern of instruction. Furthermore, the technology of prescriptive teaching and behaviorism has offered powerful alternatives to the medical-diagnostic testing model. On the other hand, cognitive-linguistic principles have provided the specific schemata and behaviors to be evaluated. Behavioristic models have given us domain referenced or criterion referenced procedures to conduct such evaluations. Current concepts provide procedures to specify levels of developmental achievement in children and to indicate the components of the equation that the child contributes to instruction.

Norm Referenced Tests Evaluation of linguistically handicapped children for too long has been based on norm referenced concepts. The original medical-diagnostic procedures evolved from the pediatric laboratories of Gesell, where child development research was predicated on the assumption that abnormal functioning could be described as a statistical deviation from the norm. Historically, this research was paralleled by the adoption of Binet's testing model for IQ to the average American school child. The movement from testing for norms of "intelligence" to norms for other domains of human behavior was a simple and logical step. Thus, the professional literature and the commercial market were overwhelmed with products to assess motor behavior, social behavior, speech behavior, and language behavior. The utility of the measurement system or test was judged primarily by its capacity to reduce complex behaviors to one descriptive term, the statistical mean for chronological age, grade, sex, and mental age.

The most fundamental error inherent in the design and structure of "language tests" is that language is conceived of as a unitary, independent human trait. "Language" is only a convenient term we use to describe a complex of behaviors organized according to levels or systems. Furthermore, it is highly dependent on the cognitive-perceptual system and is one aspect of the child's social-adaptive skills. The essential tasks in evaluating a child for language instruction are to describe the child's total level of development and to relate language skills to a comprehensive statement of development. This approach is called a criterion referenced evaluation (Turton, 1982). In this regard the clinician needs to identify the stage of cognitive development, the learning strategies available to the child, the social functions, and the sequence of development for pragmatics, semantics, syntax, morphology, and phonology.

The consistency of development across these traits is far more important than comparison to nonhandicapped age peers. Norm referenced tests are merely elaborate screening devices that identify the children who require detailed testing and the aspects of the development of an individual child that need intensive evaluation. They show who needs treatment, not the course of instruction. Without individual specification of a child's developmental level, individual instruction is simply not possible. We cannot have one without the other; to teach the child, we must know the child.

Criterion Referenced Tests Criterion referenced testing is not a new concept in language assessment. Indeed, when one rereads the original manuscript in child language research (McCarthy, 1930), the basis for significant criterion referenced procedure in language sampling can be found. Unfortunately, the prevailing concept of norms forced McCarthy to move to quantitative transformations of the data, especially mean length of response. And those who followed placed too much emphasis on this single measure of development as compared to the other scores she derived from the data. Once again, we became fixated on length, its quantification, and its mean.

A number of problems and issues related to criterion referenced testing has affected its acceptance by language clinicians. The primary reason is lack of familiarity. The beginning clinician is introduced to norm referenced testing as the only formal, acceptable system for assessment. Texts on diagnosis in speech-language pathology emphasize evaluation in terms of deviations from norms. Test administration is taught in preference to testing concepts, and interpretations are allowed only relative to tables of norms. Rarely, if ever, is the student permitted to substitute knowledge of human development or functions for descriptive statistics.

This philosophy of diagnosis creates the next major issue related to criterion referenced testing. Whereas norm referenced testing demands knowledge of a test, procedures of administration, and standardized interpretation, criterion referenced testing emphasizes a base of solid knowledge of the trait being tested. The clinician's knowledge of normal language development becomes the most important factor in assessment. The clinician must know about testing concepts (not individual tests), quantitative and qualitative modes of analysis, and interpretation relative to normal function. The stress on the knowledge base of the clinician is much greater with criterion referenced testing; thus, the stress on the academic institutions preparing clinicians is much greater. Paradoxically, the federal regulation calling for IEPs has stimulated the development of norm referenced instruments rather than criterion referenced procedures.

Often criterion referenced procedures are regarded as "informal," that is, neither reliable nor valid. This viewpoint is an unfortunate consequence of equating testing with norm referenced instruments only. Criterion referenced procedures must be reliable and valid to conform to the accepted concepts of testing. The many research studies on the reliability of language sampling are prime examples of this principle. A clinician cannot disregard the basic concepts of accuracy, stability, and consistency of scores regardless of whether the data are integrated by norms or by other pertinent criteria. The fact that criterion referenced testing requires repeated measures of a single behavior enhances its reliability.

Validity is no more difficult (or no easier) to determine with criterion referenced procedures than with norm referenced tests. It is a direct function of the relation between the items tested and normal function, between the description of the child's status of development and instructional programs. In fact, criterion referenced procedures should be even more valid than norm referenced procedures because they test functions in more depth in relation to other functions. Very simply, the concerns related to reliability and validity are false issues when applied to criterion referenced tests alone. One needs only peruse the manuals of "norm referenced tests" that argue solely for face validity to recognize how little attention has been given to these issues in our profession.

The purpose of criterion referenced testing is to specify the developmental status of the child, which we refer to here as the target population. This approach is derived directly from our knowledge of normal development. Using the framework of the Piagetian theory of normal development, the clinician can identify the stage of development (i.e., the cognitive level of development) and the specific substage. Such testing, of course, demands observation of the child interacting with and manipulating the environment. The clinician should structure the relationships between children and the objects of the environment so that each youngster has repeated opportunities to demonstrate his or her level of cognitive development.

In a similar vein, the social and pragmatic functions of the child must be catalogued as the individual interacts with the environment. Both nonverbal and vocal-verbal behaviors should be observed repeatedly to determine how children communicate their needs or desires to the environment and the relation between the style and content of communication. Regardless of which pragmatic system the clinician uses for evaluation, the essential fact is that communication follows a sequential pattern of social interaction with the environment. Formal language structures are superimposed on the cognitive-social substrata. Furthermore, there should be consistency between the child's cognitive state and the pragmatic level of development. Validity is inherent in this relationship.

The clinician must, of course, describe the language system itself. However, this description can be interpreted only in the context of the child's overall level of development because only then can the functions, content, and strategies be identified for the instructional objectives and activities of language training. If the focal point of the assessment is grammar, instruction will focus on grammar without ensuring that the prerequisites are present in the child's system. The child may be taught to use missing grammatical forms in the context of treatment, but there will not be generalization to the environment, nor will the child be able to generate similar utterances based on information present in the environment. The child will not be taught how to learn from the environment.

SPECIFICATION OF STRATEGIES OF INSTRUCTION

The recent research into cognitive-linguistic development has enriched our understanding of language forms and functions. However, from a teaching perspective, it has shown us even more about the learning process. Indeed, even without the new models of pragmatics or semantics, the research on how children learn and how they interact with the environment would have been sufficient to change our language teaching concepts. The most important message for the clinician found in this literature is that the child, from infancy on, is an *active* participant in the acquisition process. Instruction is not a set of procedures to modify the behavior of a child; it is a process directed toward helping the child to learn how to modify his or her own behavior. Cognition and language are not collections of static concepts or elements combined according to a set of predetermined commands. Nothing could be more sterile, more devoid of human reality.

The essence of the implications of cognitive-linguistic research for treatment can be summarized in a rather simple, time-honored, valid cliché. Language instruction is appropriate only when it addresses the entire complex of human development, that is, the whole child. The focal point of language instruction is not semantic-syntactic forms or pragmatic functions. The focal point of language instruction is teaching the child how to learn in the context of his or her environment. The sequence of instruction must be designed to help the child enhance the cognitive learning strategies that impinge on language acquisition.

A comprehensive language curriculum for children encompasses the three points of the developmental triad stressed repeatedly by McLean and Snyder-McLean (1978). They are the function and content of language, and the strategy of language acquisition. Typically, function (the purpose) and the content (the linguistic structure and forms) are given greater emphasis in the literature and are described in detail. Unfortunately, this arrangement distorts the normal means-end relationships of development. Function and content constitute the end products of a sequence of acquisition at any point in childhood; but, at the same time, they serve to enhance the process of continued acquisition. They are not goals in and of themselves. Adults do not speak for the sake of speaking (unless they have professorial appointments!), nor do children.

One of the most striking aspects of child development is the degree to which both the ends (function and content) and the means (strategies) can be abstracted from the sequence of cognitive development. The phases of semantic-syntactic development are intertwined with the phases of cognitive acquisition because they are interdependent on each other.

Attention

The most fundamental of all strategies is attention, the ability to focus on the relevant or salient stimulus (Hubbell, 1981). Relevance and salience can be defined only in terms of the environmental context and the purpose of a task. Stimuli to be incorporated into a child's cognitive system should be distinguished clearly from all others in the environment and should be developmentally appropriate for the child. That is, the objects cannot be determined from an adult perspective. Initially, the objects must be functional within the child's environment—items that can be manipulated and/or can impinge on the child. They must play a role in the child's life as it is structured at the time of instruction. Furthermore, the clinician must be ready to accept a minimal response, such as a gaze, a touch, or a point. The only criterion for the response is consistency. Whenever a given stimulus is presented, the child is to emit the same response.

Attention is so basic that, as clinicians, we tend to forget its importance in both the early and late stages of instruction. Unfortunately, a number of ad hoc definitions of attention now permeate the literature. Attention is not primarily a temporal function; that is, it should not be defined in terms of short or long duration. A child described as having a "short" attention span is a youngster who cannot sequence a series of attending and motor responses. The issue is not time; the issue is the child's difficulty in determining the salient stimulus in the task and shifting the focal point as the nature of the stimulus or the task shifts.

Nor should attention be defined as fixating on the human face (or "eye-to-eye contact") for a specific period of time. Except when it is an object of instruction (hence, attention), the adult human face is an irrelevant stimulus in the instructional environment. Most of the instruction will involve a horizontal gaze at objects or pictures, or an angular orientation toward a flat surface. These are the primary orientations for instruction; objects are the primary stimuli requiring attention. The motor response or activity related to the object will shape the maintenance of attention far better than a response from the adult.

The clinician must be aware that in the early stages of development, children organize their cognitive schemata according to the presence of an object, related motor tasks, and the environmental context in which the objects and activities come together. Object permanence (knowing an object is present although not in view) and early semantic forms are derived from this type of interaction. During the representational period, the child can deal with each aspect of the trio symbolically and can separate them to generate hypotheses. But until that point, the clinician must organize treatment from the perspective of the child's need to relate object to activity and to context. Without this pattern of relationships, nothing will be relevant to the child.

Matching and Imitation

Once the child has acquired the ability to attend to stimuli, the cognitive skill of matching can be introduced. Matching is the process of recognizing the similarity among objects and responding to like objects similary (Turton, 1982). The consistency of stimuli in a child's environment permits him or her to organize the relationship between objects and motor responses. The concept of matching assumes redundancy in the environment. In learning how to pattern motor movements, the child is dependent on the replicability of objects, events, and contexts. Rapid changes or different patterns constitute novel conditions and will evoke specific attending responses, but do not produce patterned relationships. Novelty must be followed by consistency to yield a patterned relationship.

As children learn similarity among objects through matching, they also learn similarity among responses through imitation. Imitation is the process of learning to *match* the responses of others to expand one's motor repertoire (Turton, 1982). Eventually, imitation becomes a procedure for learning patterns of movements and for testing hypotheses regarding one's behaviors and those of others. It is a skill available to the child to use for acquiring new responses and to perfect established patterns.

Imitation, however, does not exist as a motor skill independent of the child's cognitive-linguistic development. The degree of correspondence between the adult model and the child's response will be conditioned by the child's existing repertoire, cognitive schemata, and neuromuscular development. Children do not attempt to match for the sake of matching a response. They imitate within the context of an object and activity and their percept of the relationship between the two. The clinician must judge the degree of perfection of an imitation according to its form and the child's level of development. In particular, the imitation of a language form by children appears to be a function of its relation to their linguistic sophistication. A new form that is recognized by children and similar to their production system has a higher probability of being imitated than one already firmly established or, on the other hand, one beyond their linguistic capacity. Furthermore, the imitation of syntactic forms is possible as a consequence of a history of imitating other motor and linguistic patterns.

Discrimination

The fourth basic learning strategy is the ability to discriminate specific characteristics of objects (Turton, 1982). In the context of language, there is undue emphasis on auditory discrimination, and the child's ability to discriminate characteristics of objects through the visual field has been seriously neglected. Indeed, the latter form of discrimination is far more important to the child's differentiation of cognitive schemata. Auditory perception helps to develop the association between the object and its verbal label, but it does not have primacy over visual (or tactile) functions. Auditory labels help the child to determine the salient feature (i.e., the focal point of attention) for the discriminatory act. But, a developmental program must be designed to incorporate all forms of discrimination, varying the emphasis according to the child's developmental levels, the objects and its characteristics, the required response, and the purpose of the activity. One form of discrimination cannot be isolated for instruction without detrimental effects on others.

Relation of Child's Strategies to Instructor's Strategies

Without evidence of the presence of the four basic strategies (attention, matching, imitation, and discrimination) in a child's repertoire, instruction directed toward the functions and content of language is questionable. They are the four corners of the foundation for learning and are present throughout a person's life. As the child's level of developmental increases, the demands on these four strategies increase accordingly and so does the need for the clinician to incorporate them into the instructional format. Because a child is using agent-action-object does not mean that either cognitive or linguistic development has run its course. Many language programs fail because basic learning strategies inherent in the developmental process are disregarded. The experiential base within an environment, which is necessary for language comprehension and production, assumes that the form being taught to children has some salience for them and has been assimilated into their cognitive systems or the latter modified to accommodate the new experience. One or all of the basic strategies are necessary for assimilation or accommodation.

Specific to language, all teaching strategies can be organized under one of three headings: recognition, imitation, or spontaneous procedures. Recognition implies that we are attempting to teach a child to understand a new linguistic function or form. It assumes that evidence exists that the child has had direct experience related to the language element—that there is a prerequisite cognitive, sensory, cognitive-motor, or cognitive-linguistic substratum for the form being taught. Regardless of whether the word "boy" is being taught or the passive voice, there are experiences, schemata, and/or forms that prepare children to expand their language system. These "old forms" or "old content" must be present.

The actual strategy for teaching comprehension will vary with the language element being taught. Vocabulary is predicated on the child's cognitive schemata, which, in turn, evolve from the child's interaction with the environment. Thus, vocabulary comprehension is best taught in the context of objects and activities. In contrast, many syntactic forms such as interrogatives can be taught by using purely verbal stimuli in the comprehension task. Very simply, there is no single way to teach comprehension; there are different procedures for different language functions and forms. The important issue for the clinician is to determine the high probability strategies according to the language form being taught and the developmental level of the child.

SPECIFICATION OF OUTCOMES OF INSTRUCTION

The specification of the outcomes (attainment of goals and objectives, in IEP terminology) of language instruction is a relatively simple task when the program is sequenced in a curricular pattern. The child should be expected to show changes in function, content, and strategy. Content, in the form of number of words and number and type of sentences, has received the greatest emphasis since the appearance of generative grammar and operant procedures in the literature. This facet of language instruction is most amenable to the style of expression required in IEP statements. Most formal and informal testing procedures have focused on the measurement of vocabulary, sentence type, length of response, or production of morphological inflections. These language forms became popular in testing because they are easy to count and to convert to percentages.

There is, however, a quality of the professional functioning of speech-language clinicians that detracts even more seriously from our ability to structure a truly developmental program and to expess outcomes other than content. Unfortunately the implicit stress in our professional percept of our own behavior is on the word *speech*, not language. We view treatment as being successful and professionally appropriate only when we focus on *oral* forms of communication, only when we are talking to the child and the child talks to us. Not only have we inherited from one school of deaf education an inherent resistance to other forms of communication, we have developed our own professional bias against a sequence of objectives that stress the cognitive substrata, the functional level of pragmatics, and the processes of learning. It takes normal children approximately 6 years to acquire all aspects of language; it takes them that long to go through all three facets of language acquisition. Language instruction that ignores the importance of function and strategy is incomplete and is not developmental.

Through proper sequencing of the language instruction, the clinician can avoid this trap. At each stage of language instruction, the clinician must demonstrate that the child has acquired the necessary cognitive prerequisites, the appropriate developmental strategies, the natural social functions, and the comprehension of the language structure, as well as the expression of words, phrases, and sentences. The clinician must foster use in the treatment room, the classroom, the home, and all other appropriate environments. Language treatment must not be controlled by the mystical "80%" level of the IEP; the IEP must be adapted to the developmental process. If the clinician structures the pattern of treatment according to the natural developmental sequence, the statement of outcomes for the IEP can be lifted directly from the curriculum. But, the emphasis must be on curricular statements, not IEP criterion levels. Indeed, from a curricular-developmental perspective, the IEP can be viewed as the single greatest hindrance to progress in the art and science of language treatment because it depletes one of the clinician's greatest resources, which is time.

A language program that allots equal time and importance to the function, content, and strategies will be more successful than a content-only program because the former emphasizes teaching the child how to learn, which is the ultimate objective of language treatment. With this approach, the child will acquire the skills to cope with the environment, to learn from it, and to be independent of the clinician. The clinician who "trains" language as a series of individual elements is teaching the child to respond to isolated units only. Conversely, the clinician who expects change in all aspects of language and structures treatment from this percept is truly following a developmental model. This clinician moves from being a language trainer manipulating structures to a developmental educator fostering the acquisition of systems.

When the language clinician learns to place emphasis on all aspects of language development, the outcomes take care of themselves. The statement of terminal behaviors flows from the sequence of instruction, leads from one aspect of the triad to another, and cycles back each time. As the child acquires one level of content, the instructor learns to go back to the concept of teaching the strategy or cognitive prerequisites for the next stage of development. It is a process that has worked for normal children for millennia; it is a process that can work for the handicapped child.

SPECIFICATION OF PROCEDURES FOR EVALUATION

Because language instruction involves accepting responsibility for assisting a person through the developmental process, the clinician has a professional obligation to evaluate the curriculum. The task of evaluation is a problem of measurement; that is, to be able to answer a number of basic questions, the instructor must incorporate the most appropriate type and level of measurement into the treatment process. Whether the child has acquired the function, content, or strategy being taught is the most fundamental question. However, evaluation of instruction involves far more than the pretreatment and posttreatment testing implied in the questions relating to acquisition of a goal. This fundamental question has to be subdivided into questions regarding the prerequisites for the terminal behavior, the intermediate steps, the teaching procedures, and the problem of generalization.

Language evaluation is often divided into formal and informal testing procedures. The distinction is made on the basis of whether the procedure is a standardized test or some observation-sampling procedure. This distinction is meaningless, however, in light of the present technology of language evaluation. Very few commercially available language tests have been assessed for reliability, validity, and item analysis fully enough to warrant their being placed in the category of formal procedures. Most of the procedures available to the clinician are informal recording and observation techniques. The art of language evaluation involves knowing when to use the different procedures and how to interpret them reasonably and with caution.

The informal procedures can be placed into one of three categories: continuous recording, probes, and structured observations, particularly language sampling techniques. Each procedure has a different role in the evaluation process according to the question being asked of the data and the aspect of language being taught. The task of the clinician is to know what question to ask and how to gather the appropriate data.

Continuous Recording

Continuous recording is the recording of each response to each stimulus according to the teaching conditions. Typically, it is characterized by a correct/incorrect judgment of the child's response, made by the instructor. However, continuous recording can be utilized to provide far more information when the procedures are appropriately structured. The key issues are the design of the recording sheet and the method of interpretation. An appropriately designed instructional procedure includes a description of the element or structures being employed and the prompting procedures for facilitating correct responses. All these factors should be reflected in the data sheet so that the clinician can obtain maximum information from the data interpretation. Only in this way can the instructor know how and when to modify the instructional process. For example, when a child is not showing progress, analysis of the continuous records can tell the clinician whether the problem is the language form being taught, the strategies, or the prompts. This analysis is enhanced by comparisons with previous records, which include data on prerequisite structures, similar strategies, or similar prompts.

Continuous recording, however, does have a number of significant disadvantages. The most serious one is the amount of time required to collate all the data from a large group of children. The total number of responses must be transferred to data interpretation forms and transformed into percentages or rates of correct responses. Consequently, this form of data gathering should be reserved for two special times in the instructional process. Each time a new form or strategy is introduced, continuous records should be maintained until the child reaches the 30% correct level for unprompted responses. Then the clinician should shift to probes. The second condition that requires continuous records occurs when the child over several sessions performs without appreciable gains in the use of the language form. Continuous recording provides the clinician with the necessary data to determine whether the problem rests with the language form, the strategies, the prompts, or some yet unidentified variable.

The clinician must learn to appreciate that the percentages used in continuous recordings and probe procedures are not definitive measures of the child's language system. The percentages are merely guidelines for the clinician; they are used in making decisions about the sequence of treatment and the effectiveness of strategies. A wise clinician quickly recognizes that the criterion level specified in a recording procedure actually reflects adult behaviors and the course of treatment. The attainment of a criterion level helps the clinician to determine when to introduce new strategies or new content or to modify those in use.

Probes

For the sake of time and efficiency, probe procedures are preferred to continuous recording for most instructional conditions. A probe procedure is a sampling technique wherein the clinician obtains a limited set of data records on an intermittent basis. The only real difference between continuous records and probes is that probes are distributed in time, but data are still collected on forms for strategies, and prompts under prescribed environmental conditions. As a general rule probes provide sufficient data for evaluating instruction when gathered on a 1:4 ratio (one probe session per four treatment sessions). When the child approaches normal functioning, the probes can be spread out to 1:8 or 1:10 ratio.

Structured Observation

Traditionally, structured observation (language sampling) is the most frequently employed language assessment procedure for research purposes and one of the most infrequently used procedures in treatment. Very simply, the time involved in obtaining the corpus, transcribing the sample, and analyzing the data precludes the use of language sampling as a primary measure of success. It does, however, have an important role in validating other evaluation procedures and as a measure of generalization. Furthermore, it is the only procedure available to clinicians to evaluate the use of language forms under a variety of environmental conditions, that is, to determine the pragmatic development of the child.

Language sampling must be implemented and interpreted with extreme caution. Because it has been used extensively in developmental research, it has assumed an aura of reliability and validity. However, a careful review of the research suggests that only intraobserver and interobserver reliability of transcription has received significant attention. Test-retest reliability and validity studies are far more difficult to find and apply to evaluation of treatment. The research suggests that samples involving objects and settings other than treatment environments yield a wider variety of linguistic structures than those involving pictures and clinical settings (Longhurst and Grubb, 1974). Furthermore, a conversational-dialogue approach appears to be more productive than a question-answer format (Scott and Taylor, 1978).

The critical issue appears to be the type of measure used to analyze the transcript of the sample. Obviously, the purpose for obtaining the sample will influence the decision regarding the measures to be abstracted from the transcript. The standard developmental index is the mean length of utterance expressed in terms of words or morphemes. Both units, the morpheme and the word, yield essentially the same result. Words are preferred because they are easier to count and because they avoid the question of validating the presence of the morpheme in the child's system (Wendt, 1979).

The developmental index provides little information beyond indications that length of response has increased. It must be supplemented by data on pragmatic categories, semantic categories, and syntactic characteristics. These indices are far more significant in evaluating instruction because they reflect changes in the functional use of language, its cognitive-perceptual prerequisites, and the grammatical aspects, which the author regards as the real objectives of language curriculum. In essence, they provide more information for the clinician who wishes to make decisions regarding the appropriateness of the instructional program.

None of the evaluation procedures—continuous recordings, probes, or language samples—will be used to their fullest if they are implemented only as measures of changes in the child's language system. Evaluation of treatment implies an obligation to assess all aspects of the curriculum. To emphasize the child alone strongly suggests that the child is the only significant variable in the instructional process. In reality, the variables of curriculum design and implementation (clinician's performance) are probably far more important because they prescribe the context in which the child is expected to show changes in developmental level. Thus, an evaluation system that incorporates only formal tests and language samples to asses the child is incomplete and inadequate. A properly designed evaluation system follows the structure of the curriculum. In fact, it cannot be designed until the clinician has determined the sequence and format of instruction. An evaluation system that includes only tests and language samples is, in and of itself, an indicator that the curriculum is not designed to help the child learn how to learn because there was not proper consideration of function, content, and strategy, the developmental triad of language acquisition.

REFERENCES

Bates, E. 1976. Language and Context. Academic Press, New York.
Bloom, L., and Lahey, M. 1978. Language Development and Language Disorders. Wiley, New York.
Hubbell, R. D. 1981. Children's Language Disorders: An Integrated Approach. Prentice-Hall, Englewood Cliffs, N.J.
Liebergott, J. 1978. Assessing and facilitating communication in preschool aged children. Presentation at the Annual Convention of the Kansas Speech and Hearing Association, Wichita.
Longhurst, T. M., and Grubb, S. A. 1974. A comparison of language samples collected in four situations. Lang., Speech Hear. Serv. Schools 5:71–78.

McCarthy, D. A. 1930. The Language Development of the Preschool Child. University of Minnesota Child Welfare Monograph No. 4. University of Minnesota Press, Minneapolis.

McLean, J. E., and Snyder-McLean, L. K. 1978. A Transactional Approach to Early Language Training. Charles E. Merrill, Columbus, Ohio.

Scott, C. M., and Taylor, A. E. 1978. A comparison of home and clinic gathered language samples. J. Speech Hear. Disord. 43:482–495.

Slobin, D. 1973. Cognitive prerequisites for the development of grammar. In: C. Ferguson and D. Slobin (eds.), Studies of Child Language Development. Holt, Rinehart, and Winston, New York.

Turton, L. 1982. Communication and language intervention with severely handicapped children and youth. In: N. J. Lass, J. L. Northern, D. E. Yoder, and L. V. McReynolds (eds.), Speech, Language, and Hearing. Saunders, Philadelphia.

Turton, L. J., and Clark, M. 1971. Linguistic theory and the child. Acta Symbol. 11:42–47.

Wendt, D. K. 1979. The stability of mean length of response and mean length of utterance of the language of preschool children. Unpublished Master's thesis, University of Nebraska.

CHAPTER 6

Interactive Model for the Assessment and Treatment of the Young Child

LuVern H. Kunze, Sarah K. Lockhart,
Sharon M. Didow, and *Mary Caterson*

A model of language instruction that focuses on the prag-
matics of language teaching is presented by Kunze, Lock-
hart, Didow, and Caterson. They provide procedures for as-
sessing language and communication, and include
illustrations that demonstrate procedures for teaching com-
municative functions to young children.

1. *According to the authors, language assessment for the*
   young child should include measures of early verbal and
   nonverbal communicative behaviors. Why do they make
   this claim? What are the contexts in which the testing
   should be done? What are the measures of pragmatics
   the authors recommend?
2. *Teaching language from a pragmatic focus involves stra-*
   tegies that are largely different from those that empha-
   size syntax alone. Describe the differences. What pro-
   cedures are used when communication is the primary
   approach to language training?
3. *What is your impression of the activities used to create*
   a communicative atmosphere? Do you think they will
   help to improve the language skills of language delayed
   children?

IN RECENT YEARS THERE HAS BEEN an increased amount of information available to the specialist working with children 3 years of age and under regarding all aspects of normal development. Speech-language pathologists are more frequently being asked to diagnose and treat young children who are at the prelinguistic level of language development. The clinician has few standardized assessment tools that are appropriate for children functioning at the early stages of language development. However, recent research in prelinguistic communication (Bates et al., 1979), early pragmatic behaviors (Dore, 1975; Halliday, 1975; Snyder, 1981, Tough, 1976), and the importance of context when considering a child's utterances (Bloom and Lahey, 1978) provides a basis from which to begin assessment and treatment of young children.

This chapter describes and discusses a model of assessment and treatment for the prelinguistic and early language user. We present case examples of three children's language intervention programs that used an interactive communication mode.

Language has been described as the interaction of content (meaning), form (morphology, phonology, syntax), and use (pragmatics) (Bloom and Lahey, 1978). The same authors emphasized the interaction of cognitive growth, experience, and language use as the developmental process that results in the acquisition of language (Bloom and Lahey, 1978). The social base for acquiring language was stressed further by McLean and Snyder-McLean (1978), who concluded that communication is based largely on the early interaction of the child with the primary caregiver. We have chosen an interactive model for assessment and intervention with the very young child because it focuses on communication in a social context. Pragmatic behaviors are communicative behaviors that are used functionally in social interaction. In our model, pragmatics provides the foundation on which other early language behaviors are built.

Infants begin to affect their environment soon after birth, although this influence is generally considered to be unintentional. However, by 8 or 9 months of age, children are using gestures and/or vocalizations for intentional communicative purposes. Hence, the development of pragmatics has begun. Children continue to develop understanding of their world and later use words to code what they understand (semantics). As children begin to combine words, the semantic relationship between words in an utterance determines their linguistic word order, and semantics and syntax become inseparable (Miller, 1981). Many of the early semantic or content categories, such as agent, action, and object, are both semantic and syntactic. That is, they represent the meaning of the words and their grammatical function (Miller, 1981).

An interactive model may focus primarily on one or two areas at any given time, depending on the level of functioning and the needs of the child. For example, the child who is at the emerging one-word level will receive training that facilitates pragmatic functions and content. Another child who is combining words in many different ways will be taught to improve the form of the utterances. However, the pragmatic approach, which emphasizes communication in a natural social context, remains the basis for the assessment and treatment of language.

An interactive model provides the clinician with a dynamic context for teaching language to young children. Language treatment based on play and daily life experiences with an adult who provides modeling and expansion of the child's forms and meanings is similar to normal language learning processes. Children talk about what they know in the "here and now" (Bloom and Lahey, 1978). What they "know" is learned through play and interaction with adults. Furthermore, considering why and how children use words and gestures in the way they do increases the clinician's ability to provide the most natural and optimal situations for eliciting and teaching communication. This combination of appropriate context as well as specifically targeted behaviors facilitates maximum carryover and generalization of language skills outside the clinical environment.

This chapter examines three levels of communication development from 9 to about 36 months of age. We have selected functions described in several different pragmatic taxonomies from the work of Bates (1979), Dore (1975), Halliday (1975), Lucas (1980), Prutting (1979), Tough (1976), Uzgiris and Hunt (1975), and Westby (1980). Detailed descriptions of the various taxonomies are not given; we wish to show only the application of pragmatics to the assessment and treatment of language.

ASSESSMENT

The focus of training, particularly for the child combining words, has traditionally been on content and/or form, with less attention to systematic assessment of language use. Obviously, these are critical areas, but it has become increasingly apparent that pragmatic skills need to be included in all language assessments.

As Geffner (1981, p. 7) said, a pragmatic approach to assessment involves ". . . the interpretation of the child's utterance; the meaning intended by the child; the sensori-motor actions that precede, accompany and follow the utterance and the knowledge shared in the communication dyad.''

Standard Procedures

Our assessment of children to 36 months of age begins by applying standard tests. We view these tests as helpful in determining baseline information on salient linguistic behaviors. Examples of frequently used measures are the Sequenced Inventory of Communication Development (SICD) (Hedrick, Prather, and Tobin, 1975), the Receptive-Expressive Emergent Language Scale (REEL) (Bzoch and League, 1978), and for the young child, the Uzgiris-Hunt Scales of Psychological Development (Uzgiris and Hunt, 1975). The tests that are used to assess language functioning are not the major issue. Of greater importance is the formulation of questions about a child's communicative skills. In this regard, parents can provide important input. Just as it is important for the clinician to assess the child's use of language, it is important for the clinician to question parents, to elicit information regarding the communicative intention and use of language.

Language Sampling

The various pragmatic taxonomies in the literature force the clinician to determine the pragmatic behaviors that are most appropriate and salient for the young child. We summarize the pragmatic behaviors that are appropriate for assessment and discuss sampling methods for eliciting these behaviors.

For the 9- to 18-month-old child, our assessment includes behaviors that seem to be important prerequisites for language use. Such behaviors include tool use (the use of one object or person to obtain another object), symbolic play (child's representational abilities), object permanence (understanding that objects continue to exist, even if out of sight), use of gestures or vocalization to request, gestural and vocal imitation, communicative intent (pointing, showing, giving behaviors) and other communicative functions (e.g., labeling, calling/greeting, protesting). These behaviors have been selected from the work of Bates (1979), Dore (1975), Lucas (1980), Prutting (1980), and Westby (1980).

For the somewhat older child (18–36 months), we assess a large number of early communicative behaviors described by Tough (1976) as reporting (labeling, reporting of detail such as attributes, reporting of both present and past experiences), directing actions of self or others, and self-maintaining behaviors—the expression of wants or feelings. Also selected for assessment are communicative behaviors described by Lucas (1980) and Dore (1975). These behaviors include requesting information, acknowledgment, repeating, protesting, and responding. Table 1 describes these pragmatic behaviors.

Sampling within a pragmatic framework requires several considerations. First, the setting of this assessment should be natural, spontaneous play in which the child is encouraged to talk. Certain structured tasks may also be a part of the analysis to tap behaviors such as object permanence or tool use.

Second, the materials selected for testing should be appropriate for the child's level of cognitive functioning. For our population, we use materials that involve familiar activities and manipulative toys (Lucas, 1980). Examples of appropriate toys for the young child are dolls and layette set, tea set (silverware, plates, and cups), large blocks, pull toys, wind-up toys and, for the older child, simple storybooks, and a barn activity with farm animals.

Third, the examiner's interaction with the child should be as natural as possible. We recommend the use of nondirective statements, commenting about ongoing activities, repetition but not expansion of the child's utterances, and limited use of questions. Parents can often be helpful in facilitating the natural interaction between the child and the clinician. Above all, the clinician must be flexible. When the child does not seem to be interested in an activity, another activity should be presented to encourage communication.

Fourth, we suggest the following procedure to elicit pragmatic behaviors. An *opportunity* should be provided for certain behaviors to occur. The examiner can set up obligatory contexts that will elicit a variety of language functions (Lucas, 1980). For example, to observe the child's ability to "request objects," a situation must be established that affords the child an opportunity to ask for things.

When the desired behavior does not occur, the examiner can try to elicit it by the use of appropriate commentary (Lucas, 1980). For example, the examiner can elicit labeling by naming objects in the play setting, to establish the general idea of the task. If the behavior still does not occur, a direct *question* to elicit the desired response is appropriate.

Let's consider a child at the emerging two-word stage, noting some specific situations that can be created to observe language use, as well as content and form.

Reporting

Labeling: The examiner presents a container filled with objects and shows each one to the child, making comments such as "Look!"; if the child does not label, the examiner can make such comments as "Look! a pan!" to facilitate labeling.

Table 1. Selected communicative functions for assessment and treatment

Behavior	Description	Reference
9–18 months		
Tool use	Use of object/person to obtain another object	Bates, 1979; Prutting, 1980
Symbolic play	Child's representational abilities; pretend play	Westby, 1980
Object permanence	Child understands that objects continue to exist, even if out of sight	Uzgiris-Hunt, 1975
Request	Child requests objects, actions, either vocally or verbally	Lucas, 1980
Gestural imitation	Child imitates motor/gestural acts	Uzgiris-Hunt, 1975
Vocal imitation	Child imitates vocalizations	Uzgiris-Hunt, 1975
Communicative intent	Pointing, showing, giving behaviors	Bates, 1979
Other communicative functions	Labeling, calling/greeting, protesting, and so on	Dore, 1975
18–36 months		
Reporting		
Labeling	Child names/identifies observed phenomena	Tough, 1976; Dore, 1975
Detailing	Child describes attributes/ location of objects, actions, events	Tough, 1976
Citing present incidents	Child describes actions, events	Tough, 1976
Citing past incidents	Child describes past events (for somewhat older child)	Tough, 1976
Directing		
Others (requesting action)	Child tells listener what to do	Tough, 1976; Lucas, 1980
Self	Child's monologue, which guides his own activity	Tough, 1976
Requesting information	Child asks questions	Lucas, 1980
Self-maintaining	Child expresses wants/feelings	Tough, 1976
Requesting objects	Child indicates desired object	Tough, 1976; Lucas, 1980
Expressing feelings	Child expresses feelings	Tough, 1976
Acknowledging	Comments such as "Yeah," "Um"	Dore, 1978
Repeating	Child repeats utterances	Dore, 1975
Protesting	Child resists or denies adult's action	Dore, 1975
Calling/greeting	Child calls adult and awaits response; child greets adult/ object	Dore, 1975
Responding	Child responds to Wh-questions (e.g., what, when) and to yes/ no questions; also clarifies, agrees/disagrees	Dore, 1978

Detailing: The examiner displays two objects that are very different in size (e.g., large and small bananas or plates) and presents each separately to the child. If the child does not give detail about the objects, comments such as "Here's a little banana" may be helpful to elicit detail.

Citing Present Incidents: The examiner and the child are engaged in ongoing activities such as drinking from a cup or eating food with a spoon. Comments such as "Eat food" may help the child describe this activity.

Citing Past Incidents: Not applicable at this level.

Directing

Others: The examiner holds a bag with items in it, closed so the child will direct the examiner to open it. If this does not elicit directing, the examiner can peek into the bag excitedly to increase the child's interest and make appropriate comments as "Oh! Look what I see in the bag!" This should facilitate telling the listener what to do.

Self: The examiner observes whether the child directs his or her own actions through the use of monologues during play. If the child does not use monologues, the clinician provides language models for self-behavior.

Requesting Information: A novel object (such as a wind-up penguin toy) is placed in front of the child. The child may request information such as "What that?" The child should not be immediately shown how to operate the toy so that he or she will request this information.

Self-Maintaining

Requesting Objects: The examiner places a desired object out of the reach of the child, to get him or her to request it.

Expressing Feelings: During play, the examiner can facilitate the expression of feelings by making comments such as "Don't want egg." This behavior may encourage the child to do the same.

Acknowledging: These behaviors include the child's recognition and evaluation of responses and nonrequests. They include such behaviors as "yes," "right," and "really," and should be observed throughout the session.

Repeating: The child's repetition of the adult's utterance should also be observed throughout the session.

Protesting: To elicit protest, the examiner can put objects away before the child is finished, or do something other than what the child wants to do.

Calling/Greeting: The examiner leaves the area and reenters to elicit a greeting; to elicit calling, turn away from child, while holding desired objects.

Responding: The examiner, based on ongoing play actions, uses specific questions to obtain responding.

It is useful to have one examiner who serves as primary interactor with the child and a second examiner who serves as a recorder. In this way, the recorder is able to give feedback to the interactor regarding functions that have not yet been assessed. Also, the two adults conversing with each other and with the child create a more natural context, which should elicit the desired pragmatic behaviors.

In addition to making observations on how a child uses language, the situations can be used to assess the development of semantics and syntax. Appropriate content categories such as existence, nonexistence, or recurrence should be assessed (Bloom and Lahey, 1978), in addition to the appropriate syntactic categories.

The following brief transcript of a communicative interaction with a child at the emerging two-word stage will help the reader to understand how to apply the analysis described above. Our analysis includes the areas of content, form, and use. As the first example in Table 2 indicates, the examiner has created an obligatory content (holding a bag of objects closed) to elicit "directing." The child directs the examiner to "open." Similarly in the next example, the examiner calls attention to the objects to elicit labeling.

When language assessment has been completed, an analysis of the child's performance in the areas of content, form, and use should be made and compared with results from children of the same age to plan treatment goals.

Treatment

To implement effectively an interactive model that incorporates content, form, and use, a new orientation to language treatment is required. Heretofore, the clinician controlled the treatment program and often made the child a passive recipient. The child was rarely permitted to deviate from the pattern of behavior that was imposed on him or her to elicit language responses. In the interactive model, the clinician serves as a facilitator in a relatively unstructured program in which the child is an active participant.

Rather than constantly bombarding the child with commands and questions, the clinician comments on the child's actions at a level slightly above the child's linguistic level. This commenting is often referred to as modeling. If the adult models a variety of utterances, there is a greater chance that the child will learn the semantic rules and use of language in context rather than learning specific constructions.

Table 2. Transcription and analysis of content, form, and use[a]

Context	Utterance	Classification		
		Use	Content/Form	
E: Holds bag closed	C: "Open."	Direct others	Action	
E: Holds bag, pulls out object (cup), says "Look!"	C: "Cup."	Label	Existence	
E: Says, "Cup, yeah that's right."	C: "John cup." (as he held cup to his mother)	Label, detail	Possession in combination	
E: "Ah."	C: "Apple juice."	Label, detail	Attribute in combination	
E: "Juice, yeah"; pulls out cup, says "Sherry's cup."	C: "Mama." (as if looking for mama's cup)	Request object	Possession	
E: "Mama's cup?" "Want one for mama? Let's see"	C: "Cup, ma." (as he turns to mother)	Label + call/greet	Existence	

[a] E = examiner (Sherry), C = child (John).

We have found the hierarchy of facilitation strategies proposed by Lucas (1980) to be excellent. First, a model is provided either by a second adult or by a peer whose language skills are at a higher level. Many children respond to this model because they can observe the benefits of using language. However, some children require direct cues or prompts in the form of a question (e.g., "Who needs milk?") or instruction (e.g., "Tell me what you want."). We also use alternative question cues (e.g., "Is it hot or cold today?"), which are helpful to many children. Finally, if the child still does not respond, a direct imitation can be elicited (e.g., "Say: 'Help me.'"). We have modified these strategies to take into account the developmental level of the children and have found them to be successful.

Some other general principles adapted in part from our consultations with Sandie Barrie-Blackley and acknowledged at the end of the chapter, can serve as important guidelines for the implementation of an interactive communication program. For the young child, we advocate the following:

1. Primary focus should be on function and content initially, with a gradual shifting to work on structure as needed.
2. Emphasis should be on dialogue through integration of talking and listening (McLean and Snyder-McLean, 1978; Muma, 1980).
3. Motivating activities with participation by the child should be provided. These activities should have potential for using language in a variety of contexts (Blank, 1973; Lucas, 1980).
4. Individual needs of the child as observed by the clinician and/or reported by parents should be considered.

For the slightly older and/or higher functioning child, we also suggest:

5. The children should be guided through various activities that progress from concrete to abstract representation (Blank, Rose, and Berlin, 1978).
6. Children should be taught such key concepts as spatial relationships, sequencing, and classifying, which are relevant to cognitive development, through activities that provide the child opportunities to use these concepts in social interaction (Blank, 1973; Blank et al., 1978).

Prelinguistic and Emerging Single-Word Level

For the child who is functioning at the prelinguistic level or emerging one-word level of communicating, we use a treatment program that is largely concentrated on overall sensorimotor development with a focus on parent-child interaction. Greater emphasis is placed on facilitating tool use, symbolic play, and gestures of giving, pointing, and showing, all of which are closely related to increasing language skills (Bates,

1979; Prutting, 1980; Uzgiris, 1981). A wide range of toys is provided for the child's exploration. Pull toys, various rattles or other noise-makers, wind-up toys, and large plastic blocks provide opportunities for children to learn that they can manipulate objects and adults in their environment. Vocal and gestural exchange with the language clinician or caregiver is encouraged through sound games, pat-a-cake, and similar activities. Parents are directly involved in a number of sessions when they have the opportunity to observe the clinician as well as to participate actively. The parents are encouraged to continue these activities at home.

Case Example   K.G. is an 18-month-old boy who demonstrates delayed vocal and gestural communication development. His current communication and related cognitive abilities are characterized by:

1. An absence during vocalization of consonant sounds except for /m/.
2. Lack of emerging words or consistent sound patterns to represent objects or persons.
3. Limited spontaneous use of giving, showing, or pointing behaviors; does reach and pull.
4. Imitation of gestures, although these are limited to gestures composed of familiar schemes (e.g., claps hands, hits two blocks together).
5. Acquisition of the early stages of object permanence (e.g., successfully locates an object hidden under one screen).
6. Acquisition of early stages of tool use (e.g., pulls a towel on which a toy is placed toward himself).
7. Limited understanding of the function of objects, which is a prerequisite for the development of early symbolic play skills.

K.G. engages in limited vocal play when alone or in the presence of others. His typical means of initiating communicative interaction with others is to cry, whine, or reach to be picked up. While engaged in an activity with another person, K.G. demonstrates good attending behaviors in that he maintains eye contact as the clinician demonstrates activities. He also shows curiosity toward novel objects. K.G. does not demonstrate communicative intent either through gestures or vocalizations.

Goals and Procedures
1. *Goal*:   To increase use of communicative intentions through giving, pointing, and showing gestures.
   Task: A wind-up musical toy is operated by the adult and offered to the child. The adult verbalizes as the action is occurring, with comments such as "Here we go," "Your turn," and "All yours." When the toy ceases to operate, the adult waits for the child to initiate an action, such as returning the toy to the adult. If no action occurs, the adult reaches out and says, "Give me the toy. I'll make it go again." This response usually results in the child giving the object to the adult. Or, with an exaggerated facial expression, the adult can ask, "What happened?" The child may respond by picking up the object and either showing or giving it to the adult, who then repeats the action. The mother is encouraged to use the same strategy with the child.

2. *Goal*: To enhance early symbolic play skills through the use of object exploration and manipulation.

   Task: Common pairs of objects, such as spoon and bowl, brush and mirror, or soap and washcloth, are made available to the child. The adult comments, for example, "Let's eat!" and hands the bowl and spoon to the child. The adult waits to see how the child will manipulate the objects. If the function of an object is not clear, the child may put it in his or her mouth, throw it down, or show lack of interest in some other manner. If this occurs, the adult demonstrates the use of the objects (e.g., scoops spoonful of food out of bowl; places spoon in mouth), then hands the objects back to the child and waits to see if the child will imitate. The clinician may need to guide the child by placing the spoon in the child's hand and directing it to his or her mouth.

3. *Goal*: To pair consistent sound patterns with specific actions by using vocalizations within the child's own repertoire.

   Task: Any number of situations can be set up to include an unexpected event or mishap; for example, a battery operated toy is turned off by the adult, a toy car is rolled off the edge of the table, a jack-in-the-box toy is operated by the adult. When the toy ceases to operate or when the unexpected event occurs, the adult waits to see how the child will react. If the child vocalizes, the adult immediately imitates the child and repeats the action. When this happens a second time, the adult waits to hear the child repeat the previous vocalization and once again imitates the child. If the child does not vocalize the first time, the adult models a vocalization, such as "Uh-oh!," and encourages the child to imitate. "Uh-oh" is repeated each time the unexpected event occurs. The mother is encouraged to use this strategy in a variety of contexts, such as at meal time (should the bottle or bowl spill over the child) or during bathing (should the soap slip out of the child's hands). Other sounds can be used as well, such as the vowel /i/ during eating.

Emerging Two-Word Combinations

For the child who is beginning to combine words, we determine whether a parent-oriented individual program or a group intervention program will be most beneficial. The treatment approach is essentially the same. For those who are able to function in a group, three to five children with two adults is an ideal environment in which to encourage communication skills. Preferably, the two adults are speech-language pathologists, although a trained aide can be effective. This setting provides a situation in which many interactions between child and adult and child and child can occur. The child is able to practice what he or she is learning in a variety of ways to assure that a response does not become context specific.

We have found that a 2-hour session allows time for several different activities to be carried out, some with the entire group and some with only one or two children. Many play activities are provided, such as caring for baby dolls, play with cars and trucks, and housekeeping activities, such as cleaning and pretend cooking. These activities are geared to personal experiences to which even very young children have been exposed. Routines, such as putting on and taking off coats, snacking, cleaning up, and moving from one activity to another provide numerous obligatory contexts for using language in many ways.

When the activities do not stimulate verbalization from a child, a second adult or a higher functioning child can be helpful by appropriately modeling a verbalization. For example, at art time the top of the paste jar may be screwed on too tightly. If one child does not ask for help when needed, a second adult or another child may then model "Want help" or some other appropriate request. The first child may then verbalize a similar request as he or she observes the purpose for which language is used. If the child does not verbalize, a cue or prompt may be necessary.

Case Example   S.M. is a 21-month-old female who demonstrates mildly delayed expressive communication skills characterized by:

1. Occasional use of words with some jargon, but with very limited self-initiated verbalizations.
2. Frequent use of [∧ - ∧] with pointing and vocalization.
3. Single-word verbalizations used primarily to direct others, occasionally to label and to protest.
4. Use of existence and nonexistence content categories.

For a child of this age, we use play schemes such as cooking (tea set, silverware, pots, pans) and doll care (feeding, putting to sleep, combing hair, bathing) to facilitate obligatory contexts.

Goals and Procedures
1. *Goal*:   To use recurrence + noun (two-word combination) to request objects.
   Task: The activity involves play with a tea set, in which "pretend" juice is poured and drunk. The adult takes the pitcher from the child so that the child will request "More juice." If no request is used, the adult models "More juice" as she pretends to pour juice for the child. If a response still does not occur, the adult asks the child, "What do you want?"
2. *Goal*:   To use two-word combinations to direct others.
   Task: The activity involves having several objects with which the child needs assistance to use in play (e.g., baby bottle with cap that is difficult to get off, doll that is difficult to undress). The desired behavior is for the child to direct the adult (e.g., "Mommy off."). If a directive comment does not occur, the adult can reverse roles and model structures for the child.
3. *Goal*:   To use possessive + noun for self-maintaining purposes.
   Task: In a play activity (dolls, tea set, blocks, etc.) the adult takes an object away from the child. The child should use an utterance such as "my + noun" in attempting to take the object back. If a verbalization does not occur, the adult models this structure with other objects in the play setting (e.g., "My doll.").

Two- and Three-Word Utterance Level

Finally, as children begin using two- and three-word combinations consistently, more complex activities can be introduced. An effective activity that can be implemented in a group or individual session involves having the child make a product by cooking, art, or construction (e.g., making a toy boat) activities through a carefully planned and guided sequential process. These activities, many of which were suggested by Barrie-Blackley, are inherently motivating, are easy to individualize, provide many opportunities to practice language in a variety of ways, and can be implemented in a relatively short period of time (30–45 minutes). An additional bonus is that such activities are fun for the clinicians!

An important aspect that makes this activity different from similar activities used in many preschool classrooms is that each child makes his or her product from the first step to the last step. The child experiences the entire sequence rather than producing one step only (e.g., putting in the flour). Such activities must be carefully planned and may need to take place over two or three sessions. During the first session, vocabulary can be practiced using the actual objects for the activity, and the clinician can lead a discussion about what will be made. It is helpful to draw recipe or guide cards illustrating the sequence involved (see examples in Harms, 1981). These guide cards can then be used before, during, and after the activity. During the second session, the children actively participate in making the product. Specific concepts, structures, and uses of language are practiced, depending on the individual needs of the child. One child's goal may be to combine two or more words in making a request (e.g., "Want bread," "Want peanut butter."), while another child's goal in the same activity may be to report three of the five incidents involved in the process. We have found that a follow-up discussion involving the child and the parent is a vital component of this activity. Many children are motivated to tell their parents about something that they have made. In this regard it is usually necessary to provide the child with visual cues (e.g., guide card pictures or actual objects used) as well as auditory cues (e.g., "Did we make big or little snowmen?").

The same activities should be repeated often, so that the child becomes familiar with the vocabulary as well as the sequence involved. Language goals for the child may change with repetition of the activity, and cueing may be gradually decreased.

We have not experienced any lack of motivation even on repeated trials when the children are making play dough, toy boats, sandwich faces, and so on! These activities can then be repeated at home for further practice. We have successfully used these activities with children as young as 3 to 4 years chronologically, whose language functioning was at least one year delayed.

Case Example   C.N. is a 3-year, 3-month-old boy whose receptive language skills are normal for his age and whose expressive language is characterized by the following:

1. *Mean Length of Utterance* - 2.6 words.
2. *Content*:   Consistent use of existence, possession, recurrence, and negation; limited use of attributes, locatives, or actions.
3. *Form*:   Use of regular noun plurals; limited use of expanded verb forms such as present progressive, past tense, auxiliary, or copula verbs.
4. *Use*:   Simple reporting, most frequently labels, with occasional incidents (e.g., agent + action); use of two- to three-word utterances for self-maintaining purposes; limited use of language to direct self or others or to request information of others; no reporting of past experiences.

C.N. uses verbal language on a limited basis to interact with others, although he demonstrates adequate cognitive and prerequisite skills. He listens attentively during activities and demonstrates appropriate symbolic play skills. However, he remains generally passive in the communication process.

Goals and Procedures
1. *Goal*:   To increase three-word utterances that combine agent, action, and attributes to report incidents.
   Task: During an activity of making play dough, incidents are modeled by the two adults with utterances such as "I/we pour water," "Mash dough flat." Following this activity, the mother or peer who was not involved in the activity is introduced. C.N. uses pictured guide cards illustrating the activity and is given auditory cues as necessary to report the activity to the parent. The parents are encouraged to repeat the activity at home.
2. *Goal*:   To increase the directing function using detail such as attributes and locatives.
   Task: C.N. observes two adults or an adult and another child engage in a puzzle game. The participants alternate in telling each other where to place certain puzzle pieces (e.g., "Put big apple in," "Get little house out."). After C.N. has observed the activity for several sessions, he participates with another child. An adult provides appropriate cues as needed. Ideally, the children will gradually learn to provide each other with feedback regarding the effectiveness of the message being conveyed.

As C.N.'s language skills improved, more attention was given to form (morphology/syntax). The goals included the use of present progressive verb tense, main verb *to be*, and auxiliary verbs. These forms were taught within the interactive model because C.N. needed practice in language use and content also.

The treatment model described in this chapter is ideal for many children, but certainly not for all. For example, it may not be appropriate for children with major concomitant problems, particularly those with behavioral or emotional disorders. Children whose primary language problem is related to form, phonological and/or morphosyntactical, may not necessarily need an interactive model incorporating language use goals. An interactive model seems to be most appropriate for the low language functioning child and/or the early language user.

CONCLUSION

Normal language learning develops through the interaction of content, form, and use. Therefore, assessment and treatment for the young language impaired child should consider the purpose for which a child talks, what he means to say, and the form used to code the information (McLean and Snyder-McLean, 1978). By creating obligatory contexts to facilitate talking in a variety of ways, assessment of a young child's language abilities can occur. Treatment should then center around familiar, motivating activities in a natural context.

It is a constant challenge for the clinician to be creative when planning activities that elicit simultaneously pragmatic function, content categories, and various language forms. The clinician is rewarded, however, as the child acquires language skills at an accelerated rate and integrates these newly acquired language skills in interactions with others.

ACKNOWLEDGMENTS

The authors acknowledge Sandie Barrie-Blackley, MA, Tri-County Speech/Language Services, Elkin, North Carolina, for her contributions in treatment applications with the preschool child, and Anastasia A. Miller, MA, Duke University Medical Center, Durham, North Carolina, for her contributions in treatment with the prelinguistic child. The authors are most appreciative of their time and insight.

REFERENCES

Bates, E., Benigni, L., Bretherton, I., Camaioni, L., and Volterra, V. 1979. The Emergence of Symbols. Academic Press, New York.
Blank, M. 1973. Teaching Learning in the Preschool: A Dialogue Approach. Charles E. Merrill, Columbus, Ohio.
Blank, M., Rose, S. A., and Berlin, L. J. 1978. The Language of Learning: The Preschool Years. Grune & Stratton, New York.
Bloom, L., and Lahey, M. 1978. Language Development and Language Disorders. Wiley, New York.
Bzoch, K. R., and League, R. 1978. Assessing Language Skills in Infancy: A Handbook for the Multidimensional Analysis of Emergent Language. University Park Press, Baltimore.

Dore, J. 1975. Holophrases, speech acts, and language universals. J. Child Lang. 2:21–40.

Geffner, D. 1981. Assessment of language disorders: Linguistic and cognitive functions. Topics Lang. Disord. June:1–9.

Halliday, M. A. K. 1975. Learning How To Mean: Exploration in the Development of Language. Edward Arnold, London.

Harms, T. 1981. Cook and Learn. Addison-Wesley, Reading, Mass.

Hedrick, D., Prather, E., and Tobin, M. 1975. Sequenced Inventory of Communicative Development. University of Washington Press, Seattle.

Lucas, E. V. 1980. Semantic and Pragmatic Language Disorders: Assessment and Remediation. Aspen, Rockville, Md.

McLean, J., and Snyder-McLean, L. K. 1978. A Transactional Approach to Early Language Learning Training. Charles E. Merrill, Columbus, Ohio.

Miller, J. E. 1981. Assessing Language Production in Children: Experimental Procedures. University Park Press, Baltimore.

Muma, J. R. 1980. Language Handbook: Concepts, Assessment, Intervention. Prentice-Hall, Englewood Cliffs, N.J.

Prutting, C. 1979. Process: The action of moving forward progressively from one point to another on the way to completion. J. Speech Hear. Disord. 44:3–30.

Prutting, C. 1980. Communicative system: The model. Paper presented at the Council on Exceptional Children, Charlotte, N.C.

Snyder, L. 1981. Assessing communicative abilities in the sensori-motor period: Content and context. Topics Lang. Disord. 1:31–46.

Tough, J. 1976. Listening to Children Talking: A Guide to the Appraisal of Children's Use of Language. Ward Lock Educational, London.

Uzgiris, I. C. 1981. Experience in the social context: Imitation and play. In: R. L. Schiefelbusch, and D. Bricker, (eds.), Early Language: Acquisition and Intervention. University Park Press, Baltimore.

Uzgiris, I. C., and Hunt, J. M. 1975. Assessment in Infancy. University of Illinois Press, Urbana.

Westby, C. 1980. Assessment of cognitive and language abilities through play. Lang. Speech Hear. Serv. Schools 11:154–168.

CHAPTER 7

Creating Communicative Context

Catherine M. Constable

An important aspect of language training involves instruction in how to communicate. Constable provides a model for communication training by taking into account the relation between nonlinguistic events and linguistic events. Her illustrations show how the clinician can facilitate communication in the language delayed child.

1. *Constable introduces the terms "perceptual support" and "adapting to listener needs." What do they mean? How does Constable define these terms, and what are their implications for language training?*
2. *The phrase "clinician as communicator" is used by Constable. What is its meaning?*
3. *Constable concludes that a communicative context should have three basic components. What are they? How would you implement these three aspects of communication when working with language disordered children?*
4. *In her discussion on creating nonlinguistic support, the author introduces the terms "shared social scripts," "topic sharing," and "general event representations." Define these terms. In this regard, Constable recommends two courses of action at the beginning of language training. Find out what these are.*
5. *Examine Constable's strategies for demonstrating the use of nonlinguistic events to improve communication*

Transcriptions of clinical discourse were obtained from the Bloomsburg State College Preschool Language Nursery, which has been supported in part by Projects 451AH09072 and 029CH10044 from the U.S. Department of Education, Bureau for the Education of the Handicapped.

and language development. Do you agree with the use of these strategies? Are there others you would add?

6. *Constable discusses ways in which the clinician should use language in conjunction with nonlinguistic support. According to her, what are the values of questions, directives, expansions, imitation, and modeling? When these procedures are used, they serve a common purpose. How does the author define that purpose?*

A MAJOR ASPECT OF THE FACILITATIVE ROLE that adults play in the acquisition of language by both normal and language disordered children is the modification of the child's environment. When considering adult input to language learning, striking similarities can be found between what investigators of mother–child interaction cite as language facilitating caregiver behaviors, and what language interventionists recommend as useful clinical strategies

Bruner (1981), for example, has asserted that for normal language learners "adults artificially arrange the world so that children can do what comes naturally" and that these children "need a constrained context in order to pick up hints and cues regarding language development." Likewise, but from a language intervention perspective, Bloom and Lahey (1978) have described the interventionist as "one who manipulates the tangible aspects of the environment," whose role is to "arrange external events. . . ." Intervention from their point of view "refers to changes that are made in a child's environment for the purpose of facilitating the learning of language."

Given the semblance between what clinicians should do and what mothers of normal language learners already do, it could be concluded that to fulfill their obligation to disordered children, language clinicians simply need to replicate the input styles of mothers. This conclusion seems to have face validity but deserves further scrutiny.

For disordered children, language learning does not "come naturally" and, indeed, the character and source of deficiency may vary from child to child. Therefore, it is questionable that the undifferentiated application of a routine set of strategies that are believed to play causal roles in normal language development would suffice to meet the needs of a variety of language deficient children. Rather, it is proposed that the creation of linguistically enhancing circumstances for disordered children results from a consciously orchestrated process that has been systematized with forethought and has been individualized to meet the specific communicative competencies that the child is in the process of acquiring, while considering the nature and, perhaps, the etiology of the particular language deficit. Such a finely tuned clinical process can be developed from a general perspective of language use.

Bloom and Lahey (1978) have indicated that a basic component of language use is the influence of the nonlinguistic and linguistic contexts on the selection of alternate forms for reaching communicative goals. They propose that for speakers to devise the best form for fulfilling the function of their message, certain aspects of the linguistic context and nonlinguistic context must be considered. Figure 1 is a

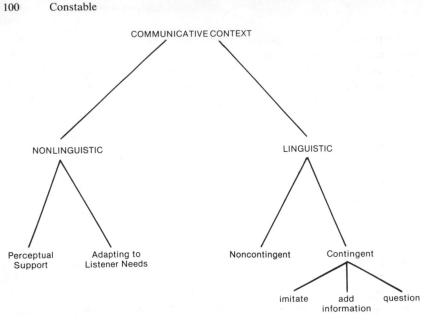

Figure 1.   Schematic representation of contextual components that affect language use. (Adapted from Bloom and Lahey, 1978, p. 19.)

schematic representation of contextual components that affect language use.

PERCEPTUAL SUPPORT

One nonlinguistic consideration in the determination of utterance form is the contextual availability of perceptual support. Before uttering a sentence, speakers must survey the nonlinguistic context to ascertain the presence or absence of referents that are related to the content being encoded in the message. If speakers discover that relevant stimuli are present, they may use this support in one of two ways. First, a speaker may direct the listener's attention to the support via pointing, gesturing, directional posturing, or some other conventional means. This direction can take place before, during, or after the generation of the speech act. We assume that the listener will make use of the perceptually available contextual information to interpret the utterance. On the other hand, the speaker, in producing the message, may assume that the listener independently will scan for and utilize available contextual information. In this case, the speaker may make no attempt to focus the listener's attention to specific context relevant stimuli.

   In the alternate condition, when there is nonexistent or negligible perceptual support for an utterance, the speaker again has two options.

One option is to alter somehow the nonlinguistic context, to create perceptual support for the utterance. The other choice is to provide linguistic compensation for reduced or absent perceptual support. Information that might have been presupposed in the event of available perceptual support must be explicitly stated. This situation often results in the use of an utterance that is semantically and syntactically complex.

The manner in which a speaker utilizes perceptual support, or compensates for the lack of it, is to a large extent determined by what the speaker knows about the listener as a communicative partner. This point brings us to the next major nonlinguistic consideration in determining the best form for fulfilling the function of the message.

ADAPTING TO LISTENER NEEDS

The content and form and function of speaker utterances are determined by several listener related criteria, the foremost being listener knowledge. One aspect of listener knowledge is general knowledge. The information the listener maintains regarding people, objects events—the world in general, for example—can guide the speaker in the generation of appropriate requests for information. Adults requesting action from very young children often point or gesture to focus the child's attention on relevant nonlinguistic stimuli. A mother who points to a ball when generating a directive such as "Get the ball" presumably does this because she has some insights into the child's knowledge (or lack of it) regarding specific lexical markers and their referents. On the other hand, preschool children direct significantly more questions to adults than to other children (Smith, 1933). This finding suggests that children consider listener knowledge to be critical to the generation of communicative intents to gain information.

A second aspect of listener knowledge is shared knowledge, that is, the amount of information that both speaker and listener maintain regarding conversational topics. To gauge appropriately the explicitness of a message, the speaker must have some sort of index for the degree of mutual understanding that exists. If, for example, the speaker knows that a particular listener is familiar with the operation of certain kerosene heaters, the formulation of an explanation for operating a slightly different type of heater probably could be accomplished verbally, by reference to the similarity to or the difference from other such devices. Here perceptual support is not necessary. On the contrary, if the speaker realizes a listener's relative ignorance of the operation of kerosene heaters, directions that are accompanied by demonstration and refer only to the basic shared knowledge of operation would probably be most successful.

Preschool children use alternate forms for conveying information about a specific event based on whether their adult listeners were present during that event. In one study (Menig-Peterson, 1975) children were more explicit and provided more information when communicating with adults who were not present during the event than with those who were. This example shows how children's presuppositions regarding shared information help them to select the appropriate form for communicating.

Another critical adaptation to listener needs is the consideration of how the listener processes information in general. The speaker may need to select alternate forms to fulfill the same communicative function for a message directed to a visually impaired listener versus a hearing impaired person. Memory, and perceptual and cognitive constraints on the intake of information, will, of course, influence the selection of input forms to listeners.

Truax and Edwards (1981) presented evidence of dramatic changes in the articulation, pitch, volume, and paralinguistic cueing of one adolescent hearing impaired reader when the composition of her listening audience as well as the function of her oral reading changed. In the first condition, the adolescent was reading aloud in an instructional exercise. A young hearing impaired child and a hearing adult were present in the treatment setting. In this condition, the reader's delivery was monotonous, unintelligible, and devoid of paralinguistic cues. When the hearing examiner left the room to respond to a phone call, the adolescent switched the function of her reading from an instructional mode to an entertaining storytelling episode for the younger hearing impaired child. With the functional switch, the reader's speech intelligibility, inflectional variance, and animation increased dramatically. No doubt this stylistic variance was a product of the reader's adaptation to the needs of a younger hearing impaired listener, as well as the alternate function of the reading episode. Other evidence regarding children's content and form changes due to sensory deficits of listeners has been presented by Schiff (1976) and Maratsos (1973).

Another way in which speakers are aided in their attempts to make appropriate presuppositions about what listeners know, or need to know, is to take into account the information exchange that has already transpired in the conversation or dialogue. And, indeed, speakers can construct conversations to provide information that the listener needs to be able to continue the topic or to interpret the speaker's consequent utterances. Therefore, consideration of the linguistic context is essential to the development of alternative forms for conveying communicative intent.

ANALYZING LINGUISTIC CONTEXT

Bloom and Lahey (1978) define the analysis of the linguistic context as the relationship of one utterance to another. Utterances within a conversational exchange may be related contingently or noncontingently. The content, form, and use of a particular speech act may, to a large extent, be based on the content, form, and intent of the utterance that preceded it. The following exchange exemplifies this phenomenon.

1. Adult A *"When do you want to go to the store?"*
2. Adult B *"How about after the football game?"*
3. Adult A *"OK."*
4. Adult B *"Will that give us enough time to get ready?"*
5. Adult A *"Yeah, I think so."*

The content of the second utterance (". . . after the football game?") was determined by the request for temporal information (signaled by the use of "when") in the first utterance. Utterances 1 and 2 are contingently related.

In the fourth utterance, the word "that" refers to a temporal entity that is not explicitly stated in utterance 3. "That" refers to a period of time that extends from after the football game (referred to in utterance 2) until the conversational partners finish "getting ready." The second speaker was able to use an indefinite pronoun form because its reference had been established, in part, within the domain of a noncontingent utterance (utterance 2).

However, it was not the linguistic context alone that was responsible for this successful discourse event. Both the speakers obviously shared information that was not explicitly stated but must have been presupposed for the communicative exchange to be successful. Such information includes the knowledge by both speakers that a trip to the store had to be made and that the speakers had to be ready for another commitment at a particular time. By appropriate consideration of the linguistic context (the utterances that composed the conversational event) and the nonlinguistic context (information the listeners shared), the communicative interaction resulted in a resolved course of future action acceptable to both partners.

CLINICIAN AS COMMUNICATOR

Communication between the language interventionist and the language disordered child is viewed here as a speaker-listener interaction designed to fulfull the language facilitation function. This function, which is to facilitate the child's ability to make inductions regarding language content, language form, and language use (see Bloom and Lahey, 1978), provides the basis for communicatively successful messages and underlies the function of all other messages the clinician directs toward the child. Once this assumption has been made, all the interventionist's alternate forms (i.e., various language facilitation strategies) can be evaluated based on how sensitively the interventionist has managed critical aspects of the linguistic and nonlinguistic contexts.

In addition to providing an impetus for self-evaluation on the part of the clinician, the notion of clinician-as-communicator has other related advantages. One of these is to keep the clinical focus on communication, thereby inhibiting the tendency of some clinicians to engage in noncommunicative "forced production drills" or apragmatic, pseudocommunicative exchanges. Second, because this perspective highlights the language interventionist's responsibility in exercising communicative competence, performance pressures that too often are placed solely on the child are likely to be reduced. Finally, the language use model (see Figure 1) provides a framework for creating a communicative context and should:

1. Provide perceptual support systems to the language facilitation effort
2. Be rich in routines, events, and materials that are familiar and adaptable to the needs of a variety of language deficient children
3. Provide a conversational structure that is natural, but specific to the goals of the participants.

The clinical application of language use principles is organized sequentially. We begin by discussing clinical management of the nonlinguistic context: the construction of perceptual support systems that contribute to the meaning and reference of both clinician and client utterances, as well as potential nonlinguistic distractors to linguistic input and output. Implications of recent research in children's acquisition of script knowledge (knowledge of the structure of routine events) and its relation to effective presupposition on the part of the interventionist precede suggestions for the construction of events that can serve as the context for intervention. We present specific examples of how linguistic input can interact with specific nonlinguistic event sequences and strategies to facilitate linguistically progressive utterances on the part of the child. Finally, an analysis of the multiple discourse functions that clinician utterances can serve within the domain of clinical conversation reveal the pragmatic application of some traditional language facilitation strategies.

Creating Nonlinguistic Support

Language is learned in the context of language use (Bates, 1976; Dore, 1979; Rees, 1978; and countless others). Therefore, a primary goal of language intervention is to create a highly communicative context, one which stimulates dialogue and conversational exchange.

According to Nelson and Gruendel (1979, 1981), the child's development of topic relevant dialogue is a function of the child's "building up of shared social scripts." That is, if children are to participate successfully in dialogic exchange, they must maintain underlying cognitive representations for events and experiences that are similar to those of the listeners. Apparently, shared knowledge of generalized event representations (scripts) supports conversational exchange and enhances communicative competence. Nelson (1982, p. 27) describes what may happen in the alternate condition:

> On the other hand, when there is no shared script, when the situation is novel, when one or both participants lack script knowledge, or when a script is not evoked (as in play with blocks or artwork), then the conversational support of the shared script will be lacking and "egocentric" speech may result.

This quotation implies that for the clinician to engage in productive clinical discourse, he or she needs to discover what the child knows about the structure of particular events and the extent of the child's knowledge regarding the roles of actors, agents, objects, actions, and attributes within routine event sequences. *Actively* seeking out an awareness of children's event representation for the specific purpose of facilitating topic sharing within the clinical setting marks a major departure from what adults normally do in an effort to communicate with children. As Nelson states (1981), "they [adults in family and school] rarely reflect upon what children's event representations are . . . and how these representations change with experience." On this basis, the clinician as a speaker needs this information to be able to make appropriate semantic and/or logical presuppositions that influence the generation of utterances directed toward the child.

Clinicians should refrain from making too many assumptions about what their clients understand about various events. Language delayed children do not always attend to the most salient features of an event, at least from an adult's perspective (Bloom and Lahey, 1978). If the clinician begins training by immediately engaging in linguistic models or questions that refer to aspects of the nonlinguistic context that have not been well established internally by the child, it can be perplexing and communicatively inhibiting for the language deficient child, particularly the hearing impaired or retarded individual.

Strategies of Intervention   Two major courses of action are recommended at the initiation of intervention. One requires determination of regular classroom and social routines in which the child is involved, and the second concerns modification of these routines. As Nelson and Gruendel remarked, "Repeated exposures lead to well known scripts" (1981, p. 29). Therefore, routine events in which the child successfully participates with a high degree of regularity are potential language facilitating activities to be replicated in language training. Activities such as brushing teeth, washing, making play dough, gathering appropriate materials for projects, birthday parties, food preparation and consumption, and classroom and household chores (e.g., washing dishes, watering plants, sharpening pencils, washing chalkboards, dusting shelves, washing windows, mixing paint, polishing shoes) are appropriate tasks for stimulating communication. The use of familiar routines as the context for facilitating progressive language use offers the language disordered child the opportunity to converse more competently outside the clinical setting. Since these routines are present in a variety of nonclinical contexts with a variety of persons, their utilization increases the probability of successful cross-context dialogic exchange on the part of the child.

The second course of action requires subtle modification of familiar routines by the clinician. The language interventionist will use familiar events or, in some cases, will introduce novel activities that utilize familiar materials. All these activities should be organized to expose clearly the sequence of subordinate structures within the event. Component processes within each activity are developed and integrated gradually, to make salient the relation between objects, actions, and actors and their operational significance to the routine.

According to Nelson and Greundel (1981), children develop a conceptual structure of a routine event as a result of observing others engaged in the routine as well as by their own participation in the routine. The language clinician provides conversational support to children by engaging them in familiar events, which give them the opportunity to observe and participate. Turn taking in this respect facilitates cognitive as well as communicative skill. A toothbrushing routine can be structured easily to enable the teaching and repetition of linguistic and nonlinguistic information. For example, if there are four language deficient children and one clinician, a tube of toothpaste can be opened and closed five different times, once for each participant. The toothpaste will be squeezed five times onto five different toothbrushes as well. Negotiation and comment regarding these processes can provide the context for the children's generation of the following target interactions:

1. To coordinate locative action or action and recurrence to give directions or comment ("Squeeze again," "Put more on this.")
2. To coordinate action with place, to give directives or comment ("Squeeze the bottom.")

As the children take turns, the component parts of the process are repeated. However, the clinician may intentionally encode the same process with two different content-form interactions. For example, both "Put the toothpaste on" and "Squeeze the toothpaste on" could be used to refer to the same event. Modeling alternate forms for encoding similar ideas is necessary for enriching children's flexibility as language users. The clinician's primary teaching objective, then, is to exploit an activity to promote language learning.

Regardless of how many times certain component parts of familiar routines are repeated and verbally marked, comprehension of linguistic input, in relationship to the nonlinguistic context, will not take place when a child does not know how to utilize perceptual support. For children with attentional deficits, "toothpaste on toothbrush" could be construed as "foot on floor" if the child fails to attend to the appropriate aspect of the nonlinguistic context. Before speaking, the clinician can use gestures to direct the child's attention to a particular aspect of the nonlinguistic context. The clinician can also demonstrate how to survey the nonlinguistic context to discern meaning. For example, the clinician may overtly scan objects, select an inappropriate referent, reject it, then pick up an object, and label it in an acknowledging manner. Similarly, this approach can be used to model a complex language interaction that involves several alternatives. For example, the clinician may tilt a pitcher saying, "Let's pour into the . . . (scan for and then select one object in an array of several) . . . cup with a handle, this one."

The number of referents, as well as their spatial organization within the clinical setting, is an important consideration. In a heterogeneous group of language deficient children, the clinician directs one child to give instructions to another. In a juice making routine, the interventionist may clear the table of all competing stimuli, provide a spoon and an open packet of juice mix to the child who does the speaking and a pitcher of water to the child who is listening. This organization of nonlinguistic elements provides perceptual support for the child's verbal response to a directive such as "Tell Jamie what to do." This particular strategy has been used to facilitate children's juxtaposition of phrases to give directions (e.g., "Pour juice in, stir round."). Again, the processes required to make juice are as important as the outcome.

Reducing perceptual support can augment the specificity of children's utterances. The following organization of events was designed to facilitate the children's use of utterances that coordinated state ("I want," "I need") and attribution ("wooden spoon," "plastic spoon") to specify or to request a desired object.

> The clinician, holding a box, confronted the children. Making certain that the children could not see inside the box, the clinician announced, "Everybody needs spoons! I have wooden spoons." (The clinician removed a wooden spoon from the box, displayed it to the children, and returned it to the box, out of the children's view.) "And I have plastic spoons." (The clinician repeated the procedure and returned the spoons to the box.) At this point, the clinician simply looked to one of the children, who initiated "I want wood spoon." This specificity on the part of the child was necessary because neither type of spoon was visually or spatially accessible.

Too often clinicians engage in questions of alternate choice. In many cases, these questions fail to elicit a complete sentence, place the client in a responder role, and can be answered nonspecifically. For example, the clinician holds two spoons, a wooden spoon and a plastic spoon, and then asks, "Do you want a wooden spoon or a plastic spoon?" to which the child could appropriately respond by pointing and saying "That one!" Typically, the clinician responds with a directive such as "Tell me, 'Want wooden spoon.'" Chapman (personal communication, 1981) cautions that this type of contingent directive may:

1. Convey to the child that there is something wrong with the appropriate use of deictic markers (a word or words for indicating or pointing to spatial or temporal aspects of a situation, i.e., "that one" in the example above)
2. Force the child to generate an utterance containing content that could be logically and appropriately presupposed (the spoons are spatially accessible to pointing and the clinician has already marked the attributes wooden and plastic; thus the child realizes that it is not necessary to specify the attributes to be communicatively successful)

To facilitate language that is rich and specific on content, the clinician must create situations in which specificity is necessary for communicative success. Structuring events with this in mind is critical to the clinical language facilitation effort.

Materials

Materials in our preschool language nursery are evaluated as appropriate if they are:

1. Present in a variety of nonclinical settings
2. Usable to demonstrate a variety of semantic relations
3. Within the motoric abilities of the clinical population

Some materials provide salient demonstration of particular targeted semantic notions but are operationally difficult. If children must concentrate primarily on how to manipulate an object, the ability to use the object for facilitating language is reduced.

**NONLINGUISTIC STRATEGIES
PREPARATORY TO SPECIFIC SPEECH ACTS**

A major goal is to increase the frequency of self-initiated language on the part of the child. Too often, clinical discourse is unbalanced with regard to interchanging of initiator and responder roles. Typically, it is the children who initiates language and the child who responds to language.

When a child initiates a communicative intent, the clinician becomes aware of what the child perceives as the important content for discussion. In turn, this information enables the clinician to make use of such language facilitation strategies as expansions and questions with greater sensitivity to the child's conversational role. Also, it is possible to construct nonlinguistic events that increase the likelihood that the child will initiate a specific speech act or attempt to code a targeted semantic-syntactic interaction. The following strategies demonstrate how nonlinguistic events can set the stage for stimulating improved language use by the child.

Strategy 1: Violation of Routine Events

Nelson (1981) has asserted that well-known scripts help children to proceed more or less automatically through event sequences:

> . . . thus freeing them from constantly attending to the ongoing action. The cognitive space so gained can be used in consideration of elements of situations that are problematic, that is, variations from routine, obstacles to completion of a goal, and negotiations between individuals engaged in an activity, (and) problem solving activities of all kinds.

When we know the nature of children's event representations, we can use this knowledge in several ways to stimulate progressive (advanced) langauge. One way is to show an *intentional violation* of routine events, for the sake of effecting a protest and/or focusing the child's attention on certain aspects of language. This strategy of violating routine events often is successful in facilitating the use of clause juxtaposition and complex sentences. Two examples of its use are provided.

Language Objective   To juxtapose clauses coding coordinate, temporal, or causal relations to give directions or comment.

Communicative Exchange   (The clinician begins to "paint" using paint powder, intentionally failing to have children mix the paint powder with water.)

1. Child$_1$: *"Hey not do the water!"* (protest/comment)
2. Child$_2$: *"Bout water?"* (request for information/action)
3. Clinician: *"Oh, I forgot to put the water in!"* (expansion/statement)
4. Child$_2$: *"Bout paint too?"* (request for information)
5. Clinician: *"Yeah, I forgot to put that water in."* (statement)
6. Child$_2$: *"Put water in, put paint in!"* (directive)

Language Objective   To code time using *and, then,* or *and then,* to describe a process or give a directive.

Communicative Exchange   (The clinician begins to turn on the blender before placing the lid on it.)

1. Client: *"No!"* (protest)
2. Clinician: *"What?"* (request for information)
3. Client: *"Put the top on."* (directive)
4. Clinician: *"Put the top on?"* (potential request for elaboration/repetition)
5. Client: *"Put top on then turn on!"* (directive)

Strategy 2: Withholding Objects and Turns

Most activities require the use of several materials, and many require turn taking. Withholding an object or turn (in an apparent oversight) is an effective method of stimulating children to initiate language to gain attention, request an object, or code intention or state.

Language Objective   To develop the use of infinitives as secondary verbs, to give directions or describe internal states.

Communicative Exchange

1. Clinician: *"Well I need a brush to paint with!"*
2. Child$_1$: *"Bout me?"*
3. Clinician: (getting brush) *"I got my brush."*
4. Child$_1$: *"Bout me, bout me brush."*
5. Child$_2$: *"Bout me."*
6. Child$_3$: *"I want it."*

7. Clinician: *"Oh, you want a brush to paint with?"* (expansion/ acknowledgment/rhetorical question) *"Here."* (hands brush)
8. Child$_1$: *"I want brush to paint."*
9. Clinician: *"Oh, you want a brush to paint too!"* *"Here."* (hands brush)
10. Child$_2$: *"I want brush paint too!"*

Strategy 3: Violation of Object Function or Object Manipulation

When children are familiar with action schemes for specific objects or object roles that compose routine events, the clinican may intentionally violate these routines to stimulate children to initiate directives and make protests.

Language Objective   To coordinate action or state with attribution, to comment, to specify desired objects, or to give directions.

Communicative Exchange   The clinician removes a large portion of paint powder from a large plastic jar, so that a long spoon is required to get the paint out of the jar. Then the clinician hands a child a $\frac{1}{4}$ teaspoon measuring spoon, $2\frac{1}{2}$ inches long.

Child: *"No, I want big spoon."*

Language Objective   To coordinate action or locative action with attribution, to describe an activity.

Communicative Exchange   The clinician holds a peanut butter jar upside down, attempting to open it.

1. Clients: *"No! . . . Not that! Hey!"*
2. Clinician: *"Not this way?"*
3. Client: *"Not that way . . . this way."* (client attempts to turn jar around)
4. Clinician: *"Do I turn the bottom part or the top part?"* (question with structure/meaning relation embedded) *"Tell me how."* (directive)
5. Client: *"Turn the top part . . . see!"*

Strategy 4: Hiding Objects

This strategy is combined with several verbal initiation strategies and has been particularly successful in facilitating development of Wh-questions and early forms for coding negation.

Language Objectives   To request information regarding location, existence, or action by using the adult form of the Wh-question; to coordinate intention with action using catenatives (linking verbs) *wanna, gonna,* and *hafta* to indicate internal state or future action.

Communicative Exchange

1. Child₁: (leaving the room to go to the bathroom) *"Watch my paint brush."*
2. Clinician: *"Hey you guys, shall we hide his paint brush? I wanna hide his paint brush."*
3. Child₂: *"I wanna hide paint brush too!"* (The children hide the brush under a chair.)
4. Child₁: (returns to the table) *"Hey, where my paint brush go?"*
5. Clinician: *"Where is it?"* (The clinician looks about the room for the paint brush.) *"Ask Brian 'Where is it?'"*
6. Child₁: (turns to Brian) *"Where is it?"*

   Language Objective   To code negation using *not, can't,* and *don't* to protest action, to describe an activity, or to comment.
   Communicative Exchange   The clinician hides the napkins.

1. Clinician: *"Jamie, you pass out the napkins."*
2. Jamie: (goes to the food box, cannot find the napkins, and returns) *"No in there."*
3. *Clinician: "Tell Patti you* can't *find the napkins."* (directive with structure/form embedded/expansions)
4. Jamie: *"Can't find!"*
5. Patti: *"Let's look on Cathy's desk."*

LINGUISTIC CONTEXT: ANALYZING
RELATION OF ONE UTTERANCE TO ANOTHER

How should language interventionists use language to fulfill the language facilitation function? A review of the literature of language development and language intervention reveals support and rejection for several mechanisms believed to play causal roles in the development of language.

   The use of questions and directives has been reported to facilitate complete constituent structure (use of the subject, the verb, and verb complement) in some normal language learning children (Bloom, Miller, and Hood, 1975). Klee and Paul (1981), however, have noted that omissions are often the correct form for answering questions in conversation. Dore (1979) has reported that the responses of younger children to questions are shorter than spontaneous descriptions and statements they produce when initiating a topic.

   Branston (1979) found that expansions contingent on children's responses to questions and models were effective in obtaining an increase in the frequency of spontaneous and imitated target structures for five language impaired youngsters. Folger and Chapman (1978) observed that the utterances that normal language learning children are most likely to "spontaneously imitate" are expansions or repetitions of their own utterances. Similar spontaneous imitations have been found to be lexically and semantically progressive, thus exemplifying the most advanced language that the child is in the process of acquiring (Bloom, Hood, and Lightbown, 1974; Moerk, 1977). It has been indicated, however, that imitation and expansion alone are not sufficient to account for the degree of linguistic competence that children usually acquire (Brown and Bellugi-Klima, 1964).

Miller and Yoder (1974) and Bricker, Dennison, and Bricker (1976) have advocated the use of elicited imitation and modeling as procedures for language training. Courtright and Courtright (1976, p. 656), however, introduced some partial opposition to the use of elicited imitation by stating that ". . . requiring an immediate response to a stimulus can disrupt the retention process by not allowing sufficient time for coding to take place." This controversy in the literature regarding the role of imitation in both normal and disordered language acquisition could be due in part to the lack of explicit differentiation among and between the various types of imitation being investigated (see Prutting and Connolly, 1976).

The use of modeling can increase sentence length and complexity in both monolingual and bilingual children (Harris and Hassemer, 1972). Modeling has also been found to lead to the transfer of newly learned grammatical structures from use in one situation to use in another (Carrol, Rosenthal, and Brysh, 1973). Leonard (1975) noted that the association between what is being modeled and the events of the nonlinguistic context must be made salient to the child if successful modeling is to be effected. These "events of the nonlinguistic context" are never explicitly outlined by Leonard. This omission is unfortunate because the degree to which perceptual support and paralinguistic cues affect linguistic events is presumably high (Bransford and Nitsch, 1978; Labov and Franshel, 1977). However, some interventionists (Longhurst and Riechle, 1975) emphasize situational support and describe various interactional routines that provide children with the opportunity to use the language they are learning.

Perhaps, to analyze successfully the teaching efficacy of modeling, expansion, and elicited imitation, the procedures need to be studied and evaluated as communicative events. The author contends that the success of a particular strategy cannot be determined without studying its function in a specific conversational domain.

Analyses of video- and audiotaped transcriptions have indicated that verbal strategies often can serve a variety of discourse functions depending on the conversation. An expansion, for example, can function as an acknowledgment in one conversation and as a request for clarification in another conversation. Furthermore, it is evident that verbal language facilitation strategies can serve more than one discourse function in a conversation just as ordinary speech acts do. It is beyond the scope of this chapter to treat the discourse functions of all possible language facilitation strategies; however, four have been selected for discussion: elicited imitation, expansion, modeling, and questions.

For many clinicians, there is an undeniable attraction to the use of elicited imitation as a language facilitation strategy, yet some recommend this strategy be used only *if all else fails* (Bloom and Lahey, 1978). The author believes that with planning, clinicians can create situations wherein elicited imitation can be used to facilitate children's utterances that are: (1) communicative, (2) pragmatically appropriate, (3) fulfilling of the child's communicative intent, and (4) linguistically progressive. The following transcript is offered for analysis.

Language Objective

Child₁: To request information regarding location, existence, or action by using the adult form of Wh-questions.

Child₂: To coordinate intention with action using catenatives *wanna, gonna,* and *hafta* to indicate internal state or future action.

Communicative Exchange

1. Child₁: (leaving the room to go to the bathroom) *"Watch my paint brush."*
2. Clinician: (to other children) *"Hey you guys, should we hide his paint brush?"*
3. Clinician: *"I wanna hide his paint brush."*
4. Child₂: *"I wanna hide brush too!"* The children hide the brush under child₃'s chair.)
5. Child₂: (returns to table) *"Hey! Where my paint brush go?"*
6. Clinician: *"Where is it?"* (clinician demonstrates searching behavior)
7. Clinician: *"Ask Brian, 'Where is it?'"*
8. Child₁: (turns to child₃) *"Where is it?"*
9. Child₃: *"Here under this, my chair."*

According to Chapman's (1981) levels of analysis, at the "utterance level" the communicative function of utterance 6 is a request for information. At the "discourse level, utterance related" (how the utterance functions in relation to an utterance that immediately precedes or follows it), utterance 6 is an expansion of the utterance that immediately precedes it. It continues the topic of the conversation and also provides a model that is preparatory to the directive in utterance 7.

The use of the elicited imitation strategy in utterance 7 stimulated the child to use an adult Wh-question form, which was communicative, pragmatic, fulfilling of the child's original intent, and linguistically progressive in that the copula "is" was used by the child in utterance 8. Here the clinical goal was to teach language form. Thus, when the clinician gave the directive to use an adult Wh-question (Where is it?), she reduced the semantic complexity of the model by dropping out the possession relation (my) and reduced the utterance length by deleting "paint brush go" (see utterance 5). This change could be made because reference to the paintbrush, with the pronoun "it," had been established by the contingent relationship of utterance 6 to utterance 5. The meaning relation was likewise indicated by the clinician's display of searching behavior. Furthermore, the child was directed to communicate his intent to a listener who maintained the requested information and was willing and able to respond.

A universally advocated strategy for verbal language facilitation is "modeling" (McLean and Snyder-McLean, 1978; Bloom and Lahey, 1978; Courtright and Courtright, 1976). To provide a model, it is recommended that clinicians map their language onto the action of the child using semantic-syntactic interactions that are sometimes reduced in length and complexity and reflect the clinical goals of the child (Bloom and Lahey, 1978). Presumably, this strategy will stimulate the children to talk about their own actions and states (Bloom and Lahey, 1978). A close look at this strategy raises some questions. Although the semantic-syntactic character of the utterance may be appropriate to the child's activity, it must be emphasized that whenever the clinician talks about what the child is doing, the clinician is providing a model of how language is to be used and, in this case, how to use language to talk about what *someone else* is doing. Furthermore, once the clinician has encoded information about the child's action, that information becomes old. To encourage or demand that the child consequently encode the same information merely stimulates children to communicate redundant information. The motivational aspect of this exercise is questionable. However, if the clinician replicates the child's activity and then comments on this activity, a model of how to comment on one's own activity has been generated.

The following two examples demonstrate modeling in a sequence in which the clinician observes the child's activity, replicates it, and generates a comment to refer to her own action. In these instances, the children followed with spontaneous comments.

Example 1   The child is painting a piece of Styrofoam, which causes a scratching noise.

Clinician: (begins scratching her paint brush against her Styrofoam)
             "Hey Amy, hear me painting?"
Child₁: (spontaneously looks to Amy) *"Hear me paint, Amy?"*

Example 2   All children have received paint cups and are awaiting paint.

Clinician: (holds up her paint cup) *"Look, I have a white paint cup."*
Child₁: (holds up paint cup) *"I have black paint cup."*
Child₂: (holds up paint cup) *"I have white cup!"*

The use of vocatives ("Hey Amy!") and notice imperatives ("Look!") clearly mark the communicative nature of the models.

Expansions of children's utterances refer to the generation of a contingent utterance that syntactically completes the structure of the original utterance (Muma, 1971). Expatiations refer to contingently generated utterances that increase the semantic content of the original utterances. Expansion and expatiation can be used therapeutically without disrupting the flow of conversation because these strategies can function simultaneously as other speech acts.

Language Objective   To develop coordination of locative action with possession in two or three constituent utterances, to comment, to give a direction, or to specify location.

Communicative Exchange

1. Clinician: *"What do I do?"* (holding up a bottle of glue)
2. Client₁: *"Put it on."*
3. Clinician: *"Put it on my paper?"*
4. Client₁: *"No, put on my paper."*

At the "utterance level," utterance 3 functions as a potential request for elaboration (see Garvey, 1979). At the "discourse level, utterance related," utterance 3 functions as an expansion, to continue topic and also as a model preparatory to utterance 4.

If clinicians become aware of the multiple discourse function that language units can fulfill, these strategies can be used without disrupting the continuity of the conversation. Indeed, with some forethought and practice, clinicians can "get the most from their messages."

A similar analysis of utterance 1 of the last example reveals an additional level of discourse function. Using the Chapman (1981) outline, utterance 1 is analyzed as follows.

1. Utterance level: requests information.
2. Discourse level, utterance related: initiates topic.
3. Discourse level, speech act related (the function of utterance in relation to the total conversation): in this situation, the clinician uses the question to prepare for the use of an expansion of the child's forthcoming utterance.

In this example, the clinician's first strategy was intentionally preparatory to her second strategy. The clinician used the question to initiate a series of conversational turns that would eventually lead to a linguistically progressive utterance on the part of the child.

This illustration demonstrates that questions do not always need to be ends in and of themselves. Questions can be used to initiate topic or to parcel out small bits of information that can consequently be expanded on. Also, questions can stimulate children to seek out information, as in the following example.

Clinician: (to Brian) *"Where's Trevor's cup?"*
Brian: (to Trevor) *"Where you cup?"*

The instructional use of questions (eliciting an answer to something the speaker already knows) can be overused by clinicians. A sensitive clinician realizes that instructional questions are not the only communicative forms for gaining information from the child. Focusing children's attention on the absence of materials from familiar places can stimulate children's initiation of information regarding the whereabouts of objects:

Clinician: (pointing to the easel where a rainbow had been) *"Our rainbow! . . ."*
Child: (running up to easel) *"Here rainbow under this!"*
Clinician: *"Oh, our rainbow was hiding under the squares!"*

Simply stimulating children to attend to novel objects or actions offers them the opportunity to be initiators rather than responders:

Clinician: (pointing to a worm) *"Look at that!"*
Child: *"That moving on there! See, go go go."*

CONCLUSION

It is proposed that situations give rise to the effective application of various language intervention strategies. That applicability is context dependent. Devising the best form for fulfilling the language facilitation function requires that the interventionist integrate, often simultaneously, all relevant information from the communicative context. Such spontaneity requires a functional awareness of the various ways that routine events, paralinguistic cues, perceptual support, and the language objectives of the child can interact with the multiple discourse functions of clinician-client utterances. This awareness is functional to the extent that it stimulates the clinician to begin effecting interactions between linguistic and nonlinguistic events to create contexts that enhance the child's communicative skills.

ACKNOWLEDGMENTS

The author thanks Laureen Leffkowitz Curry for her insights into the development of this chapter. Thanks also to Judith Hirshfeld, Julia Weitz, and Jean Yoder for editorial remarks on an earlier version of this chapter.

REFERENCES

Bates, E. 1976. Language in Context. Academic Press, New York.

Blank, M., Rose, S., and Berlin, L. 1979. The Language of Learning. Grune & Stratton, New York.

Bloom, L., and Lahey, M. 1978. Language Development and Language Disorders. Wiley, New York.

Bloom, L., Hood, L., and Lightbown, P. 1974. Imitation in language development: If, when, and why. Cog. Psychol. 6:380–420.

Bloom, L., Miller, P., and Hood, L. 1975. Variation and reduction as aspects of competence in language development. In: A. Bick (ed.), Minnesota Symposium on Child Psychology, Vol. 9. University of Minnesota Press, Minneapolis.

Bransford, J. D., and Nitsch, K. 1978. Coming to understand things. In: J. F. Kavanaugh and W. Strange (eds.), Speech and Language in the Laboratory, School, and Clinic. MIT Press, Cambridge, Mass.

Branston, M. 1979. The effect of increased expansions on the acquisition of semantic structures in young developmentally delayed children: A training study. Unpublished doctoral dissertation. University of Wisconsin.

Bricker, D., Dennison, L., and Bricker, W. 1976. A language intervention program for the developmentally young. Children with Communicative Disorders Monograph Series, no. 1, Mailman Center for Child Development, University of Miami.

Brown, R., and Bellugi-Klima, U. 1964. Three processes in the child's acquisition of syntax. Harvard Educ. Rev. 34(2):133–151.

Bruner, J. 1981. The social context of language acquisition. Keynote address at the Sixth Annual Boston University Conference on Language Development.

Carrol, W. R., Rosenthal, T. L., and Brysh, C. G. 1973. Social transmission of grammatical parameters. J. Educ. Psychol. 63:589–596.

Chapman, R. S. 1981. Exploring children's communicative intents. In: J. F. Miller (ed.), Assessing Language Production in Children: Experimental Procedures. Vol. I. University Park Press, Baltimore.

Courtright, M., and Courtright, I. 1976. Imitative modeling as a theoretical base for instructing language disordered children. J. Speech Hear. Res. 19:655–663.

Dore, J. 1979. Conversation in preschool language development. In: P. Fletcher and M. Garman (eds.), Language Acquisition. Cambridge University Press, Cambridge.

Folger, J. P., and Chapman, R. S. 1978. A pragmatic analysis of spontaneous imitations. J. Child Lang. 5:25–38.

Garvey, C. 1979. Contingent queries and their relation in discourse. In: E. Ochs and B. Schieffel (eds.), Developmental Pragmatics. Academic Press, New York.

Harris, M. B., and Hassemer, W. G. 1972. Some factors affecting the complexity of children's sentences: The effects of modeling, age, sex, and bilingualism. J. Exp. Child Psychol. 13:447–455.

Klee, T., and Paul, R. 1981. A comparison of six structural analysis procedures. In: J. F. Miller (ed.), Assessing Language Production in Children: Experimental Procedures. Vol. I, p. 88. University Park Press, Baltimore.

Labov, W., and Franshel, D. 1977. Therapeutic Discourse. Academic Press, New York.

Leonard, L. B. 1975. Relational meaning and the facilitation of slow learning in children's language. Am. J. Ment. Defic. 80:180–185.

Longhurst, T. M., and Riechle, J. E. 1975. The applied communication game: A comment on Muma's "Communication game: Dump and play." J. Speech Hear. Disord. 40:3.

Maratsos, M. 1973. Nonegocentric communicative abilities in preschool children. Child Dev. 44:697–700.

McLean, J., and Snyder-McLean, L. K. 1978. A Transactional Approach to Early Language Training. Charles E. Merrill, Columbus, Ohio.

Menig-Peterson, C. 1975. The modification of communicative behavior in preschool-aged children as a function of the listener's perspective. Child Dev. 6:1015–1018.

Miller, J., and Yoder, D. 1974. An ontogenetic language teaching strategy for retarded children. In: R. Schiefelbusch and L. Lloyd (eds.), Language Perspectives–Acquisition, Retardation, and Intervention. University Park Press, Baltimore.

Moerk, E. 1977 Processes and products of imitation: Evidence that imitation is progressive. J. Psycholinguist. Res. 6:187–202.

Muma, J. 1971. Language intervention: Ten techniques. Lang. Speech Hear. Serv. Schools 5:7–17.

Nelson, K. 1981. Social cognition in a script framework. Working paper, City University of New York.

Nelson, K., and Gruendel, J. 1979. At morning it is lunchtime: A scriptal view of children's dialogues. Discourse Processes 2:73–94.

Nelson, K., and Gruendel, J. 1982. Generalized event representation: Basic building blocks of cognitive development. In: A. Brown and M. Lamb (eds.), Advances in Developmental Psychology. Lawrence Erlbaum Associates, Hillsdale, N.J.

Prutting, P., and Connolly, J. 1976. Imitation: A closer look. J. Speech Hear. Disord. 41:3.

Rees, M. 1978. Pragmatics of language. In: R. Schiefelbusch (ed.), Bases of Language Intervention. University Park Press, Baltimore.

Schiff, M., 1976. The development of form and meaning in the language of hearing children of deaf parents. Unpublished doctoral dissertation. Columbia University, New York.

Smith, M. 1933. The influence of age, sex, and situation on the frequency, form, and function of questions asked by preschool children. Child Dev. 4:201–213.

Truax, R., and Edwards, A. B. 1981. Reading as a language process. Workshop presented by the Alexander Graham Bell Association, White Plains, N.Y.

CHAPTER 8

Facilitating Language in Emotionally Handicapped Children

Amy Belkin

Treating emotionally handicapped children with language disorders is a demanding but fullfilling experience. Belkin tells how she works with these children and describes the procedures and techniques she uses.

1. *Belkin uses the term "facilitation" when describing her language treatment procedures. What does this term imply to you? Do you regard it as synonymous with "intervention and training"?*
2. *The term "working alliance" is employed by Belkin to describe the relation between the clinician and the emotionally disturbed child. What does this term mean? How is a working alliance implemented? Do you agree with Belkin as to its importance?*
3. *Describe Belkin's language training model for the emotionally handicapped child. What linguistic concepts are involved? How are developmental concepts utilized?*
4. *What pointers has Belkin provided for language assessment? What are four contexts for sampling the language behavior of children? What analysis is made of the language responses?*

Masculine pronouns are used throughout this chapter for the sake of grammatical uniformity and simplicity. They are not meant to be preferential or discriminatory.

The children described in this chapter were enrolled in schools for the emotionally handicapped. That is, a certified psychiatrist or psychologist had diagnosed each one as having a severe emotional handicap. A variety of psychiatric disorders are usually found in such schools, including childhood schizophrenia, autism, and severe character disorders. The children's names and ages have been changed to protect their identity.

5. *In setting up a program of language training, Belkin lists several basic goals. What are they? Do you agree with her? Additionally, Belkin discusses five techniques to facilitate language. What are they? Would you use these techniques? Do you recommend other techniques?*

6. *From your understanding of this chapter, do you think the methods and procedures for treating language disordered children should be different depending on whether the children are emotionally disturbed?*

For most of each day, Lisa, a 4-year-old autistic girl, stood in the middle of the small classroom shaking a piece of torn paper. She watched it through the corners of her eyes as a tense grimace distorted her beautiful face. She was apparently unaware of the teachers and other children, who went about the business of learning and relating to each other. What was so compelling about shaking paper? Why was Lisa so untouched by all the emotions and experiences that we find to be the very essence of life? How should we teach meaningful, spontaneous language to such a child? Where to start?

Facilitating language acquisition in emotionally handicapped children is one of the most demanding, soul-searching, yet fulfilling experiences in a speech-language pathologist's career. Moreover, this experience is continuously evolving as we learn about each new child with his unique constellation of psychodynamic, perceptual, cognitive, and linguistic symptoms. For language cannot be investigated or taught in isolation, separate from a child's other problems.

Emotionally handicapped children do not sit dutifully as we go about the business of teaching language. If ever there was relevance to the tenet "Teach the whole child," it applies to these children. They confront us fully with distress and confusion and we must address these issues within each child and within ourselves if we are to know them, and if we are to teach them.

WE START WITH OURSELVES

Establishing a working alliance with an emotionally handicapped child requires emotional responsibility and personal investment. It is essential to project full appreciation of each child's unquestionable worth regardless of his young age and numerous problems. Such respect is crucial for the child's growth and is essential for establishing and maintaining a working alliance.

Well and good, but hard to do when the child is unresponsive, bites for no apparent reason, or undermines every language activity you present. In a school for emotionally handicapped children these experiences may be everyday occurrences. Here, too, a special kind of emotional responsibility comes into play. Now I'm not talking about realizing that he's a child and you're an adult and you're going to pull yourself up by your professional boot straps and rise above it. This concept implies that you have resolved not to be emotionally affected by the child's behavior. If your student is a biter, continuously calls you "ugly" or "mean," and refuses to participate in treatment, you *will* be affected!

Psychiatrists describe an emotionally handicapped child's behavior as reflecting his transference of earlier feelings for "significant adults" onto another adult—you. For example, a child may be frustrated in his attempts to achieve emotional fulfillment from his parents. He's going to make sure you feel that frustration as well. He's going to undermine your attempts to teach him by demonstrating hatred of your activities and materials or by subtly showing resistance, such as complying with every language task but never learning.

Your reaction will probably be a combination of several emotions—such as frustration, guilt ("What am I doing wrong?" "What made me think I could teach anyway?"), and anger. And here's the rub. Psychiatrists suggest that we not ignore our feelings, but tune into them as truthfully as we can. Our own feelings can often act as a mirror showing us how a child feels. When he makes you feel totally incapable of teaching him, its not because of poor lesson planning; rather, it's because he feels incapable of succeeding, and he needs to let you know. Treatment has to start there—in facilitating the child's sense of being in control, of having successes and experiencing fulfillment with a caring adult. Whether language tasks are continued or temporarily put aside is up to you. The main issue is that recognition of your own reactions has become a sensitive and essential tool for knowing that child and how to teach him.

Probably most of us have been taught to write "Establish rapport" as an initial goal of the first clinical session. It can become a pat phrase that may not take on full significance regarding the complexity of the task until you've spent many months in accomplishing that one goal, so that the child is ready to learn.

You will need to be extremely flexible to meet best the learning needs of each emotionally handicapped child. This ability can be achieved if you have incorporated a model of language development and facilitation firmly in your mind. With this internalized foundation you will be able to assess and encourage language in the variety of settings in which emotionally handicapped children are taught.

My first job was a vivid example of this need. I was the speech-language pathologist at a therapeutic nursery in New York City. Before starting I was given two rules. First, children could not be taken out for individual or group training while school was in session, because leaving the classroom and separating from teachers and other children might create anxiety. Second, I was not allowed to bring materials into the room, especially materials that were designed for one child, because the other children might become jealous.

I was a guest in someone else's classroom. In those early months my role was secondary to that of the teachers. They created and choreographed all classroom activities, and I facilitated language growth when and where I could. To walk into a classroom with no procedures of my own and no materials in hand, and yet to be responsible for teaching language, I had to have firmly defined goals consistent with established principles of language acquisition for each child. Yet I had to be flexible on any particular day.

USING BLOOM AND LAHEY'S MODEL

The model of language facilitation that I find most valuable when teaching children at these early stages of language acquisition was developed by Bloom and Lahey (1978). Their treatment plan embraces the three major components of language—content, form, and use—without which propositional, communicative language would not be possible. *Content* refers to concepts about people, animals, and objects, as well as to actions, events, and processes. *Form* consists of the conventional systems of speech sounds, words, and syntax. *Use* includes the variety of purposes for which language is intended. All three components are integrated within each utterance. That is, every utterance we speak embraces meaning, displays some level of form, and is spoken for a particular purpose. A treatment plan must address all three components of language to be successful. The Bloom-Lahey model does just that.

Normal Language Development

Bloom and Lahey base their language training plan on normal acquisition of cognitive and linguistic processes. In the normal development of the child, there are stages of interrelated social, perceptual, cognitive, and linguistic growth. These interdependent domains must show development before successful progression to the next stage is possible. Therefore, Bloom and Lahey recommend that language skills be taught in a sequential order consistent with normal growth. In terms of the content of an utterance, for example, we would begin by helping the child code the content categories that develop early, such as the existence of objects, and their disappearance and subsequent recurrence. Only after these and other early content categories have been used in the child's spontaneous language would we encourage the acquisition of more sophisticated meanings, such as causal relations between events, coordination of two objects, and time.

Intervention based on the sequence of normal development involves not only language, but also social, perceptual, and/or cognitive domains. For example, autistic children, functioning at a delayed perceptual-cognitive level, frequently demonstrate fascination with minuscule configurations of objects, such as a crack in a table or a piece of dirt on a window pane. These preoccupations with meaningless bits of information will not assist the children in building concepts of tables or windows nor in acquiring the labels and functional terms that communicate these concepts. In such cases I have found it effective to promote sensorimotor growth as an initial goal while facilitating the ability to communicate through words and phrases. Hence, knowledge of the sequence of normal development helps us in knowing what to teach and in what order.

Understanding Children's Language Disorders

Another value of the Bloom-Lahey model is that it is sufficiently comprehensive to address the range of language problems exhibited by emotionally handicapped children. For these children, every component of language may be delayed or disordered.

Disorders of Content   Emotionally handicapped children often exhibit disorders in acquiring and expressing various content categories. These disorders can be due to a delay in perceptual-cognitive development. For example, Robby did not express through language two types of negative meaning, namely, the disappearance and nonexistence of objects. Moreover, he rarely asked for an object or person that was not in view or for an event that had been completed. The content categories of disappearance and nonexistence are dependent on a child's ability to perceive, integrate, and maintain images in specific contexts. Subsequently, the child must recognize and integrate the absence of the person or object in that context and either signal this absence or request its reappearance. Robby's lack of expression of these meanings, coupled with his nonverbal behaviors, reflected weakness in these abilities. It is consistent that Robby did not represent one object for another in play, nor did he refer to events in the future or in the past.

In addition to perceptual and cognitive deficiencies, psychodynamic disorders may preclude the use of content categories. The following example illustrates this point. Although his general linguistic ability was well within normal limits, Ralph did not reject the unacceptable actions of others. Instead, he expressed distress by running away, whimpering, crying, and pointing in the direction of the stressful context. Ralph's inability to communicate rejection verbally reflected his difficulty in expressing such emotions. His psychotherapist afforded insight into the problem. For Ralph, negative words "could kill," therefore, he would not use them at any cost. Inability to express rejection was not easily overcome in spite of the verbal modeling, encouragement, and support of Ralph's teachers and psychotherapist.

This example highlights the importance of knowing all aspects of an emotionally handicapped child's problems. Such a task is best achieved through participation in all case conferences, reading reports, and maintaining an open dialogue with teachers and psychiatrists. In Ralph's case it was important that the clinician not encourage utterances signaling rejection until negative words were no longer imbued with heightened emotional content.

Disorders of Form   Disorders of form are also apparent in some emotionally handicapped children. On one level this deficiency may be observed in problems identifying and producing speech sounds, and in using prosodic features. For example, Suzanna's verbal abilities were difficult to observe because of her poor intelligibility, rapid rate of production, loud intensity, and relatively high pitched tone. These behaviors seemed to reflect a frenetic, emotionally charged communicative style. Another behavior that occasionally gave Suzanna's language a bizarre quality was her use of klang associations. At such times she appeared bound to repeat speech sounds or words produced in the preceding utterance. While playing with another child she said:

> What a nice time/
> One time/
> What a night/

Finally, Suzanna produced utterances that appeared to reflect her inability to maintain a stable memory for speech sounds or sequences of sounds necessary for producing words. The following example reflects her apparent attempt to produce the name "Kevin." Beckoning to Kevin to play, she said:

> Hey Ka/
> Here Kitty/
> Come on i Kin/
> Come here Kevin/

Disorders of form also include the inability to retrieve words. I have frequently observed this problem in emotionally handicapped, language disordered children. Because of his many other language problems, Paul had not yet found a compensatory strategy for his severe word retrieval problem, such as talking around the forgotten word or substituting another term, which would have allowed him to continue communicating. Rather, as soon as he realized that he could not retrieve a word within the sentence he had begun, he started speaking through clenched teeth and reduced the level of his voice until his words were inaudible. Eventually he refused to talk.

Difficulty in acquiring rules for syntactic structures is the most frequent disorder of form experienced by these children. Six-year-old

Jessica, for example, knew about objects and events, which she readily attempted to communicate through a variety of uses, but she had difficulty learning words and rules for combining words. Jessica, in her teacher's arms, not wanting to leave the swimming pool said:

No leave/

Emotionally handicapped children also exhibit breakdown in form as it interacts with content and use. The autistic child's preoccupation with the raw, perceptual configuration of speech sounds, devoid of meaning, is a type of echolalia that reflects this breakdown in form. For example, 9-year-old Peter could imitate with exact pronunciation, intonation, and pauses songs previously heard on records. On one occasion he imitated a song until he came to a place where the record had been cracked. Like the recorded version, Peter continued to repeat the words exactly as they had been distorted by the crack until his amazed teachers intervened. He seemed to make no distinction nor to show preference when echoing meaningful versus distorted words.

Disorders of Use   Disorders of use are also prevalent in emotionally handicapped children and are characterized by a range of symptoms and varying degrees of severity. Here is an example of a severe deficit in use. Jenny, a 6-year-old autistic child, did not respond verbally or with gesture to attempts by others to engage her, nor did she initiate communication. She was silent during the nursery day with only two exceptions: on occasion, Jenny echoed the teacher's utterance with exact vocal inflection, and, when fearing a favorite toy would be taken away, she pleaded for it by rapidly calling its name in a high pitched, monotone voice. Jenny had been overheard privately using single- and two-word utterances. However, for purposes of communication she was electively mute.

Some children talk about events that are out of context. Twelve-year-old Lester, greeted everyone with an involved description of yesterday's news. He spoke spontaneously with appropriate syntax and accurate knowledge of the content of the news. However, he rarely spoke about events in the immediate context or attended to subjects that were interesting to others.

Some children assume that the listener knows their thoughts and previous experiences. They cannot take the listener's lack of knowledge into consideration. Wes, a 12-year-old emotionally disturbed and hearing handicapped boy, referred to events that had occurred the previous summer, substituting the pronouns *he* and *she* for names, and *it* for objects. When the teacher asked questions to clarify what actually had happened Wes became enraged, insisting that she really knew but was trying to provoke him.

One additional symptom of a disorder of use is the emotionally handicapped child's inability to recognize the underlying implications of utterances. Thirteen-year-old Dan reached the corner ahead of his classmates. His teacher reminded him to look both ways before crossing the street. Dutifully, he did just that: he looked up and down the street, but then walked into the path of a moving car (which successfully swerved to miss him). The unspoken reason underlying the teacher's request had been unrecognized. Dan, like many other emotionally handicapped children, could comprehend only the literal meaning of a statement. Such incidents are dramatic examples of just how literal and restricted that comprehension can be!

These descriptions are far from inclusive. However, they suggest the value of relating this range of diverse language behaviors to a cohesive and comprehensive model. In my experience the majority of young, emotionally handicapped children exhibit moderate to severe delay affecting all domains: psychodynamic, perceptual, cognitive, and linguistic. In terms of language, even if these children present symptoms of language disorder—such as klang expressions, excessive echolalia, word-retrieval difficulties, elective mutism, prosodic disturbances—they also exhibit delayed language. And it is this delayed language that can ultimately form the basis for subsequent language growth.

Although I attempt to enhance social, perceptual, and cognitive skills, my major effort as a speech-language pathologist is to facilitate growth in language. I have found that I can teach children to code content categories, to acquire through induction rules of syntax, and to expand through experience their knowledge of use, all of which are critical components of learning how to communicate.

Assessment

Before writing treatment goals, we must amass sufficient information to determine the child's language system. However, we cannot study this knowledge directly. The child cannot explain his rule system any more than the average adult can describe all the grammatical rules he uses. In addition, the child may be cognitively or emotionally unable to participate in formal testing. Hence, we must discover this knowledge indirectly.

The most effective approach I have found is to observe children in natural settings. In the child's school, the classroom and the playground afford an opportunity to observe his general behavior and language in an environment in which spontaneous, informal communication between children and teachers is encouraged, and toys, furniture, and objects are freely manipulated by children.

It is essential to observe social, perceptual, and cognitive skills because problems in these domains may provide cues to why language has not progressed normally. In each domain the list of behaviors to observe is lengthy. Here are just a few examples.

Assessing Social Skills   Does the child make eye contact, seek comfort from others, and seem to be aware of teachers and classmates? Can he attend to class activities, or instead, does he stimulate himself by making sounds, rubbing hands or feet over surfaces, rocking back and forth, or becoming rigid because of some internal excitement? Does he relate to other children only by physically attacking them for no apparent reason? Does he separate from his mother and teachers without recognition that they have gone? Does he scream or withdraw when anyone other than his primary teacher approaches? Interference with the normal development of interpersonal relations, as evidenced in the latter behaviors, may herald additional problems, augmenting the value and purposes that verbal communication serves.

Assessing Perceptual Skills   Assess the child's gross and fine motor coordination as a reflection of physical maturation. Note whether the child characteristically smells and tastes objects as a developmentally early means of learning about them. Informally observe whether the child is hypersensitive to sound. Some children grimace in pain and cover their ears when spoken to at normal level. A similar hypersensitivity may be noted for light. Observe the child's ability to see and hear individually and in combination. Autistic children, for example, do not always use these distance senses of vision and audition even when they have no problem with acuity. Jeremy illustrates this problem. Outside school he never seemed to look where he was going. He characteristically tilted his head to one side. He ran in bursts, first up the sidewalk, around in circles, almost into a building, then practically into the street. Jeremy and I were good friends. On one occasion I bent down to greet him as he charged toward me. Without looking he swerved around and started down the street. However, when I called he did a double take and quickly came into my outstretched arms.

Even when autistic children use the "distance" senses, they may not demonstrate this ability beyond a limited circumference of say, several feet. This perceptual deficiency gives the autistic child the appearance of being in his own world, unaware of and unaffected by the environment around him. Additionally, autistic children may not use their senses in combination. Thus, they may not localize to the source of a sound. Eight-year-old Paul was engrossed in playing with a paint brush. To his teacher's amazement, he made no response when a piercingly loud fire alarm abruptly began clanging nearby.

Assessing Cognitive Skills   There are numerous cognitive skills to observe. Does the child understand what he is expected to do during class activities? Can he postpone manipulating an object but instead observe and learn from another's handling of the object? Does the child's behavior indicate that he has acquired the concept of object permanence—that absent objects continue to exist? Does he show the ability to represent one object for another? Can he appreciate cause-and effect relations in his manipulation of objects? The importance of such behaviors in fostering early language development must not be underestimated. For example, one early developing skill is the ability to follow visually the direction of another's finger, pointed to an object, person, or event. Underlying this gesture is the child's acquired awareness that the focus of attention, the object pointed to, should be shared by himself and the person pointing. Autistic children may not have acquired this aspect of appreciating another's reference. Envision the cognitive and language development that is missed by the child who never looks where a parent, teacher, or classmate is pointing.

Assessing Linguistic Skills   In assessing language production, we need to observe three types of interrelated information: 1) the child's exact utterance; 2) utterances spoken by teachers and other children before and after the child speaks; and 3) relevant nonverbal context. Because the same utterance can mean different things, depending on the context in which it occurs, these data are essential for making the most accurate interpretation of the concepts underlying the utterance, the form used, and the communicative intent.

The child's ability to comprehend language must also be assessed. Although a full portrayal may not be possible during observation of spontaneous behavior, the child's responses to literal and implied commands, direct and indirect questions, and comments are noted. Receptive language is more thoroughly investigated through predesigned tasks and formal tests.

We are interested in developing as valid a picture of the child's current language skills as possible, to distinguish language skills that are characteristic of the child's present level from occasional behaviors. To achieve this goal, both the length and the variety of the sample must be considered.

I take a 2-hour sample at the beginning of each school year. Even this sample does not represent all language behaviors of the child. So I supplement it by taking minisamples designed to tap expressive behaviors and receptive skills that may not have occurred. For the sake of variety, each 2-hour sample is divided so that the child is observed in at least four different contexts: 1) in semistructured lessons, such as cooking, and in free play; 2) when happy, and when distressed; 3) when needing to communicate and when content to be alone; and 4) when in a group and when with one other child.

Ideally, both written and taped transcripts are used. Taped transcripts are essential for capturing entire conversations, especially when children talk quickly and in complex sentences. Unfortunately, the level of ambient noise in an active classroom can easily drown out taped utterances. Hence, when in class, I take as complete a written transcript as possible to supplement the taped recording.

Interpretation

Next the interpretive work begins. It is necessary to assess the presence or absence of each content category, the level of structure, all contexts in which language is used, and the variety of purposes that language serves. Make an interpretation of the meaning of each utterance, based on verbal and nonverbal descriptions. For the most part, it is easy to interpret children's referents from their utterances because young children usually comment about objects and events in their immediate environment. Except for delayed imitations, and utterances based on internal images or hallucinations, this method of analysis holds true for the majority of utterances spoken by emotionally handicapped children. That is, from the situation or context, the clinician can interpret the content category referred to by the child: The teacher requests that 8-year-old Andrea sit in her chair: "Go sit down." Andrea, sliding to the floor, said "No." This utterance was interpreted as rejection of an unwanted event that directly affected Andrea. Also observe whether the child coordinates several content categories in one sentence to form more sophisticated meanings. For example, Brian coordinated the existence of objects with possession. When referring to a doll's bed, he said "That's her bed."

Regarding form, observe the child's articulation skills, vocal resonance, and intonational patterns. I have known numerous emotionally handicapped children who had hypernasality, a voice pitched too high, monotonous intonation pattern, and a rapid rate of speech. Observe the range of vocabulary. For example, there may be word substitutions and an abundance of pronouns in lieu of nouns, which may indicate difficulty in word retrieval. Calculate the mean length of uttterance as well as range of utterance length. Note the presence of major sentence constitutents, subject and predicate, as well as inflectional endings, such as *ing* or *ed*. Observe the variety of the sentence structures— questions, negatives, imperative statements, compound and complex structures, and so forth.

In assessing communicative use, note the contexts in which the child speaks. For example, does he always echo utterances spoken by others? Does he initiate conversation or only respond to others? Can he build a conversation or does he use one utterance per topic? Interpret the function that each utterance, verbal and prosodic, serves (e.g., to direct, request, assert). Note whether the child speaks only about personal needs (this is true of many emotionally handicapped children) or whether he can refer objectively to events in the environment. Then evaluate how these three components of language interact. That is, determine whether there is an effective integration between the purpose (use) for which each meaning (content category) is communicated by words and sentence structure (form).

Next, note the frequency of each content category, form, and use. Language skills that are regarded as productive are those that occur in a number of different instances within the 2 hour sample. Also note which skills are absent, or present but not productive. Finally, determine how social, perceptual, and cognitive skills support or hinder language growth.

GOALS

My goals are to facilitate the acquisition of approximately six absent or emerging receptive and expressive skills that occur early in the normal sequence. For example, at the single- and two-word utterance stages, most children talk about the existence, disappearance, recurrence, and rejection of objects and events, in addition to actions and actions that change the location of objects. If absent, these relations are chosen as initial goals for treatment because they are the easiest for the child to identify and learn; also, subsequent language development is based on their having been acquired. Hence, the child may learn to request (use) the recurrence of objects (content category) using single- and two-word utterances (form). When the children demonstrate acquisition of these relations in their spontaneous behavior, new goals are chosen from absent or emerging language skills in the next stage of development, and so forth.

CURRICULUM AND PROCEDURES

The curriculum for language teaching in young, emotionally handicapped children is basically the same as that for other children with delayed language. Each interaction between content, form, and use becomes a theme, and the children are given numerous opportunities to induce these relations and, subsequently, to use them. Content, form, and use relations can be facilitated by participating in cooking, creative movement, story time, listening to records, and play with representational objects. These are standard teaching activities in preschool classrooms. As an example, a child who is learning to understand and express actions that affect the location of objects might be exposed to numerous events in which objects and people change place.

For the clinician who works in the classroom, this procedure can be accomplished easily in individual and group language training sessions. A trip to the playground is full of locative action events. Clinician and child can comment on sand being dug up and poured into pails, bottles, buckets, sieves, and cups. Similarly, sand can be poured out only to be scooped up again. Children can request turns swinging backward and forward, up and down. They can call attention to themselves as they slide down and climb up the sliding pond or while on the jungle gym. Even games of hide and seek can be turned into language lessons exploring how locatives can be coded into words. Back in the classroom, there are numerous opportunities to listen and to express locative action events. Activities such as making vegetable soup stimulate locative action utterances because they include scraping off carrot peels, putting cut up vegetables in the pot, pouring liquid into the pot, stirring it around, and watching the steam rise and so forth.

Establishing a Working Alliance

Emotionally handicapped children's special needs create obstacles for using the materials and activities mentioned above in addition to learning language. Finding the most effective means of overcoming these obstacles becomes a major procedural issue. The following discussion focuses on ways of minimizing the learning problems of these children.

Developing a working alliance starts when we first meet the child. We may be immediately confronted with behaviors that interfere with our ability to establish rapport. For example, Marshall was uncommonly fearful of adults other than his primary teacher. When someone looked directly at him, he either froze in place or gasped loudly, and turned away while shuddering with fear.

Children like Marshall must determine the extent to which they can tolerate the presence of another person, and I have learned to tune into the child's pace of accepting a new relationship. Imposing yourself on a child, even in a positive and friendly manner, may cause the child to back away. The need to identify and adopt to the child's pace also applies to language stimulation. Alan's teacher was intent on describing the picture he was drawing in spite of the boy's growing tension. The teacher encouraged Alan to label various objects and persisted in asking him numerous questions. The vocabulary level, sentence structure, and concepts were appropriate for a nursery school child, but Alan could not tolerate the unending onslaught of words. He finally screamed for the teacher to stop talking, and put his head on his desk. The teacher sat back, confused. She had considered only a preconceived idea of language stimulation, and had not been sensitive to the amount of language this particular child could process at any one time.

In the early weeks of school, I usually start by coming into the classroom during free play, sitting near the new child, and watching him work. Sometimes I comment on what he's doing or encourage his efforts. How directly I interact with the child depends on how much he can handle. Eventually he will allow me to join his activity.

However, his trust of me may not develop easily. In this regard other children are enormously helpful. Most of the new child's classmates relate warmly to me because they were in language treatment the previous year. They show their enthusiasm in coming to "Amy's room." Finally, their active participation in group sessions enables the new child to see what's expected of him. At this point participation in group activities may not be possible. Participation isn't forced. Rather, there is always a place set aside for the child, and he is reinforced with verbal praise and smiles for attending as he views the group activity from a distance. For the new child who is not ready to be taken for individual treatment, I do individual work in the classroom while the teacher is working with the other children.

Techniques Used to Facilitate Language

The child hears sequences of speech sounds while interacting with the environment. He has to develop rules regarding how concepts extracted from the environment and sequences of speech sounds go together. A primary task in language training is to establish the most effective environment for this process to take place. I recommend the following procedures for facilitating language growth: mapping, modeling and expanding utterances, eliciting language, and encouraging feedback skills. These five procedures are easily incorporated into informal, relatively spontaneous verbal interaction in the classroom as well as in structured individual and group training sessions.

Mapping   In this symbolic process, sequences of speech sounds or gestures represent an object or event. Mapping is the first step toward language development, and I have known several children who, upon recognizing this correspondence, have experienced a burst of language growth. The key to mapping language is to make the correspondence between the event and the word as vivid as possible. I choose the most relevant single words and use them with emphasis as the child engages in an activity. Since you never know when the mo-

ment of realization will occur, it pays to encourage spontaneous repetition of words. Six-year-old Eddie occasionally used single words but
they were mostly inappropriate to the situation. One fall morning Eddie
was using the sliding pond. As he slid down I said "slide" and "down"
loudly and with falling intonation. "Climb" and "up" accompanied
his climbing the stairs and "again" as he ran around to start his climb.
Eddie began to listen, and our game continued for 10 minutes. If I
hesitated he would wait for me to say "up" before beginning to climb.
The following day I lifted another child in Eddie's class and said "Mel-
inda up." Eddie turned around smiling. He chanted "up, down, up,
down" all the way to the playground. By spring he was speaking in
simple, complete sentences, and was referring to events in the past
and future. I believe this growth began at the sliding pond when he
realized that words map events.

Modeling   The technique of modeling consists of providing for a
child a component of language that he does not use or uses marginally.
The clinician, for example, can model content categories. Signaling
recurrence is a category that can be modeled by saying "more," while
giving the child additional juice at snack time or flour while making
play dough. In terms of form, the modeled utterance incorporates only
one linguistic element beyond the child's habitual utterance length.
That is, for Juan who habitually produced single-word utterances, I
modeled two- and, at most, three-word utterances. The modeled utterances never extend much beyond a child's expressive level of language because it has been my observation that most children demonstrate an equally restrictive utterance length for understanding language. Providing utterances that are slightly in advance of those used
by the child is a way to highlight the relationship between content,
form, and use without taxing comprehension. Finally, the clinician can
model the uses of language. In a previous example we saw that Ralph's
teacher modeled "No" to prove to the child that he could use negative
utterances without the words actually causing physical harm to the
other child. Alan had a severe deficiency in knowing how to use language. He initiated language only in the form of a question. Through
modeling, other ways of communicating were demonstrated, such as
giving directions, requesting information, and calling attention to himself.

My inclination is to employ modeling as an activity is taking place
and, if the children remain focused on the task, I model again after the
event. Young emotionally handicapped children cannot postpone manipulating an object that is the focus of their attention. These are not
the children to wait their turn to stir the cookie dough. Therefore,
unless the modeling is immediate, you lose their attention. Moreover,

for many young children, language input that precedes an activity is not particularly helpful. For example, before drawing a picture of the members of their family, these children may derive no benefit from giving the names of each family member. Rather, for them the action must lead the language experience. Each child must be an active participant in an activity for language to become a meaningful part of the relationship.

A word about repeating the same activities. Because of perceptual and cognitive disabilities, many emotionally handicapped children need repeated experiences. Only after complete exploration of the motoric and perceptual structure of a task can a child acquire mental representations about the objects and actions within the event. Without these mental representations he will be unable to attend to the language that maps these events. Hence, although I offer children a variety of activities for learning content-form-use relations, I feel justified in repeating activities

Task repetition is also essential from a psychological point of view. Some children anticipate failure when they are presented with a new, unexplored activity. Repeating the event enables the child to observe the requirements of the task. With familiarity, the original fear may diminish and the child may subsequently be able to participate. One thing to look out for, however, is the child who creates stereotyped responses out of original, spontaneous action. For such children, repetition of tasks can become ritualistic behavior.

Expansion   A form of modeling, expansion consists of paraphrasing the child's utterances to include an additional developmentally appropriate content-form-use relation. For example, at juice time the child might say "more." If you realize that the child wants juice, expand on his utterance by saying "more juice" and then help the child produce this utterance to his teacher. The teacher in turn can demonstrate greater comprehension of the two-word utterance: "Oh *now* I understand. More juice! Of course you can have more juice," said in a way that is tailored to the child's level of comprehension. Hence, expanding the utterance helps the child get the results he wants. He needs to communicate, and you're giving him the words.

For children with limited language skills, I begin with major constituents. For example, if a child produced a verb as a single-word action, I would subsequently expand it to "action-affected object" or "agent-action."

I always try to make the relation between utterance and event as vivid as possible. Paul, for example, signaled action-affected object relations ("Sit chair"), but never incorporated the agent of the action into these structures. To make this salient, I emphasized the linguistic form during each event in which Paul participated. As we took walks, for example, I would model two- and three-word utterances that included us both as actors: "Paul run," "Amy run," "Paul fall down," "Amy sit down," "Paul stop," "Amy stop," and so forth. What is vivid for the child, not necessarily for you, must be considered. Each time we went back to his classroom, David, a 5-year-old autistic boy who spoke in single words, put his eyes next to a crack in the wall and slowly moved along the wall, keeping close attention to the length of the crack. I also touched the crack, named it, and showed him other cracks, which I coded with the content categories *existence* and *recurrence*, as in "another crack," and *action*, as in "touch crack," respectively. In this manner, David's preoccupation with perceptual configurations, such as lines and lights, became a vehicle for demonstrating that I appreciated what was of interest to him and for helping him associate these figural preoccupations with linguistic form.

However, psychodynamic problems can hinder a child's ability to focus objectively on materials. Without being able to establish a mutual reality, there is no way to use mapping, modeling, and expanding techniques effectively. Seven-year-old Ronnie imbued objects with the virtues of "good" or "bad," and "beautiful" or "ugly." Involvement with this emotional content interfered with his ability to focus on language tasks. For example, when we worked on color identification, Ronnie saw orange as "good" and purple as "bad." He reacted to the presence of these colors with pleasure and disgust, respectively. He could not focus objectively on the color of objects and consequently failed to learn their names. This emotionally based learning disability reached serious proportions when Ronnie projected his personal reality onto almost every material he encountered. What was reality for him was interfering with the implementation of appropriate language goals. When this is the fundamental issue, psychiatric care is recommended. Moreover, a psychiatrist could offer supervision to the language pathologist to optimize the potential for language learning.

Eliciting   Encouraging the expressive use of language, by direct and indirect teaching techniques is called "eliciting." Direct techniques involve creating specific activities that encourage the expression of particular content-form-use relations. Indirect teaching involves creating everyday classroom situations where the utterance is used to establish a positive outcome (Lucas, 1980, p. 213). Frequently, methods change as the child's learning needs progress. That is, when the child is ready to generalize a new linguistic skill, the teaching mode frequently changes from using direct to indirect methods. For example, one goal that was set for 10-year-old Bobby was to learn to request objects. After he could express this function in individual treatment, his teacher gave him the job of handing out lunch boxes. First, however, she hid several lunch boxes, so that Bobby had to ask for them to complete his job.

One value of group training sessions is to encourage children to talk to each other, because the activities are child oriented rather than adult oriented. Adult oriented interactions occur when each child's utterance is directed back to the clinician, who remains in constant control of the communicative interaction. I use both direct and indirect methods to encourage child oriented interactions. Child-to-child inter- action can be fostered by direct teaching. For example, instructing Jennifer to "Tell him 'stop,'" or "Say 'no,'" was necessary to assist her in rejecting the hurtful embraces of other children. Children com- municating with children can also be encouraged through indirect meth- ods. For example, having the children rearrange the furniture will give them time to explore the various uses of language as a means of gaining cooperation to accomplish a task.

Feedback   Feedback becomes useful when a working alliance has been established, and the child demonstrates beginning competence in integrating content, form, and use, for example, in producing one- and two-word utterances. Feedback techniques incorporate modeling, ex- panding, and eliciting. Here the goal is to provide certain cues that can assist the child in becoming sensitive to his own language product and in being able to compare his language with the model language. There are a number of ways to implement feedback cues and a number of considerations to keep in mind (Lee, Koenigsknecht, and Mulhern, 1975, pp. 18–23). For example, expanding a child's utterance to the next developmental level and requesting him to imitate the expansion is a procedure in which maximal cues are provided. In contrast, saying a word that the child omitted is an illustration of giving a minimal cue; in this case the child is responsible for incorporating the word correctly. Requesting spontaneous expansion of an utterance requires even more responsibility; this technique is used only when the child has given evidence that he can produce the utterance.

In another feedback technique that I have used successfully, se- verely language disordered children analyze their own utterances. Evan, an autistic 9-year-old boy, spoke in rapid, unintelligible phrases. His poor comprehension and pat utterances indicated that he had learned whole phrases, almost as envelopes of sound, but had not yet identified the individual words or their interrelation. My goal was to increase Evan's identification of individual constituents and their re- lation within each sentence. Evan's primary modality was visual, so I began writing down everything that Evan said. Even intonational pat- terns were schematized by writing up and down the page to make the connection between his speech product and the written word as vivid as possible. Phrases and words were then slowly read back to Evan, and I helped him add words he had omitted. This procedure enabled him to isolate specific words because his usual rapid pronunciation of whole sentences could be broken down into meaningful components. Through such activities Evan's spontaneous expression of sentence structure became longer. Evan's identification of the components of language did not stop at the word level but resulted in fascination with speech sounds. He spontaneously began to play with sounds while I wrote them down. He would repeat one sound a dozen times, then change to another. It seemed that in addition to going forward, we had gone back to the beginning of language, and, at 9 years of age, Evan had begun to babble for the first time.

One feedback technique I regard to be an important procedure in language training involves the selection of the appropriate sensory modalities for optimal language learning. The ultimate goal is for each child to be able to use all modalities and, whenever possible, the auditory-vocal channel for language. The modalities to which each child best responds are initially used for language training. For 5-year-old Eric, initial selection of the appropriate sensory modalities for input appeared to be crucial. Consequently, during the initial stages of training, language tasks were shifted from one modality to another as a means of reducing perceptual fatigue. At the same time, perceptual activities were used to increased Eric's ability to perceive, discriminate, associate, and tolerate auditory information and, later, information across modalities.

The manner of stimulus presentation will maximize the child's success for receiving information. Having Tim put his hands in his lap reduced random arm flapping and helped him to attend calmly to an activity. Presenting few, well-separated stimuli, putting materials at the far end of the table (to decrease the child's impulse to grab them), and repeating instructions were helpful in keeping Tim on task.

Selecting the appropriate means of responding is equally important. For example, when sorting pictures into categories, Tim placed them on each pile in random trial-and-error fashion. The perceptual excitement of waving the pictures in the air appeared to distract his attention. However, asking him to point to the correct category before being given the picture resulted in 100% accuracy.

The rate of presentation must also be taken into account. Pacing affected Howie's ability to participate in activities. When I spoke in a quiet, gently modulated voice, using a relatively slow paced presentation, Howie appeared transfixed. He would stare into my eyes, his face and body immobilized. Howie had trouble maintaining personal boundaries and a slow paced, quiet lesson seemed to merge his boundaries with mine. In contrast, vivid, action based tasks of give and take, which were presented at a fast pace and with a high level of enthusiasm, seemed to foster successful interaction and accurate performance.

THE WAY IT LOOKS ISN'T ALWAYS THE WAY IT FEELS

We started our discussion by saying that recognizing a child's need to make you feel the way he feels and your use of this information is an important part of successful work with emotionally handicapped children. Frequently, the way the child acts "on the surface" may not represent the real message he is trying to convey.

Charlie always wanted to be first to leave his class for individual instruction, but this was not always possible. On one spring day, waiting was just too much. "Why can't you take me now? I want to go with you," he whined, as I brought each child back to his room. Assurances that Charlie would be going soon were to no avail. His complaints reached a crescendo of anger and tears. After trying to console him, I had to leave the room. After all, there *was* a schedule to keep and other children waiting. Sobbing, Charlie followed me to the top of the stairs. "Damn you, Amy, damn you!", he bellowed until his teacher retrieved him. The assistant director met me at the bottom. With a wise smile he asked, "And why is Charlie damning you today?" This time the answer was easy: "It was a sign of love."

ACKNOWLEDGMENTS

The author gratefully acknowledges the encouragement, support, and helpful suggestions of Prof. Margaret Lahey, Institute for Health Science, Hunter College, City University of New York, Susan Diamond, speech-language pathologist for the Reece School, New York; and her husband, Marvin Belkin. Fond thanks are also offered to Alice Childs, Director of the Reece School, and Dr. Robert Miller, Consulting Psychiatrist to the Reece School, for sharing generously of their time and knowledge.

This chapter is dedicated to the memory of my father, Bernie Stone, with appreciation and love.

REFERENCES

Bloom, L., and Lahey, M. 1978. Language Development and Language Disorders. Wiley, New York.

Lee, L. L., Koenigsknecht, R. A., and Mulhern, S. 1975. Interactive Language Development Teaching. Northwestern University Press, Evanston, Ill.

Lucas, E. V. 1980. Semantic and Pragmatic Language Disorders: Assessment and Remediation. Aspen, Rockville, Md.

CHAPTER 9

Language and the Atmosphere of Delight

R. McCrae Cochrane

Cochrane considers ways to encourage spontaneity of language in aphasic patients. She advances the position that undue emphasis on the conscious control of speech will inhibit the spontaneous use of language, and, therefore, can inhibit the retrieval of language.

1. *What does Cochrane mean by "the atmosphere of delight"? What are its objectives?*
2. *How does Cochrane define spontaneous language? In this regard, what is meant by learning a language through conscious awareness? According to Cochrane, what procedures can be used with aphasic patients to teach language without conscious awareness? What are some training procedures that inhibit the retrieval of the spontaneous use of language?*
3. *Sometimes a clinician wishes to focus on deviant grammatical forms that occur repeatedly. What approaches can be used that do not adversely affect the development of spontaneity in the use of language?*

IN PAST CENTURIES, PARENTS must have sensed the importance of the enchanting moment when a child takes his or her first steps alone, for families created their own celebration of the occasion long before pediatricians and researchers invested it with the status of a developmental milestone. As parents become aware of their child's increasing readiness, they even attempt to create the opportunity by conspiring together: one parent lets go of the child's hands as the other calls invitingly for him to come. With one of my own children this event was particularly memorable.

It occurred on a neighborhood playground. My daughter was around 12 months old, at the stage when she edged around the furniture in a standing position. She was always careful to reach out for the object ahead before moving forward, but when speedy arrival was important, her confidence returned her to earth, where she could crawl comfortably. One afternoon she was alone, comfortably messing around in the dirt, when she spotted a large black dog entering the play yard. Her reaction suggested the unexpected presence of a famous dignitary. "Goggie!" she exclaimed with delight. Her eyes widened, and she rose up, stretching her arms out wide. "Goggie! Goggie!" She had taken 11 steps before it dawned on her that she had done something new!

This experience may illuminate for us some aspects of the natural learning process and also reveal some interesting implications for language remediation. First, the experience took place naturally and spontaneously. Certainly it could not have occurred without both the child's readiness and the particular event that served as its catalyst. However, no adult had said "Look at the dog!" or "Take 11 steps," or "Say 'dog.'" Thus, a directive figure (teacher or parent) was not central in determining the action during the moment the new behavior emerged.

Second, the child was so immersed in her response to the situation that her first steps were accomplished without any conscious awareness, much as we all usually walk. In fact, the conscious realization of what she was doing finally halted her, as though she had suddenly remembered she was not able to do what she was in fact doing.

Third, obvious delight and interest were precursors to the spontaneity of the behavior. For whatever reason, the focus was definitely on the *dog,* rather than on the task of accomplishing a word or a step. Walking, talking, and gesturing all occurred within the environment of her delighted interest.

Fourth, the moment belonged entirely and personally to the child. Certainly it may have been related to previous parental encouragement, but at that moment I was out of sight on the other side of the yard. The moment engaged her cognitive apparatus, her motivation, her physical readiness, her emotional release, and her own unique pattern of self-expression. If you and I were given the same idea to express verbally, the chance that we would produce identical sentences would be extremely slim. Language contains shared patterns, but it is a personalized system of expression.

Fifth, the spontaneous verbalization "Goggie!" was inseparable from the flow of the entire reaction. The scene exhibited cognitive, linguistic, gestural, emotional, and physical components, but these were inextricably tied to one another within the reality of that moment. Even the verbalization "Goggie" conveyed more than the ability for referential object identification. My daughter's voice expressed the joy of recognition and the anticipation of pleasure, and these messages were wedded to her existing cognitive and linguistic frame.

SPONTANEOUS LANGUAGE

This chapter examines how conscious awareness, self-expression, and ongoing experience affect spontaneous language, and explores their use for intervention in language acquisition and retrieval. In so doing, I present some thoughts about a new clinical direction, an emphasis on the disciplined and systematic development of a particular atmosphere as a conscious treatment strategy. Ideally, this atmosphere would function in a way similar to what was observed in my daughter's first steps. In defining this strategy, I propose the term "the atmosphere of delight," which means the overall clinical objective geared toward enhancing spontaneous communication. Then I explore how such an atmosphere can relate importantly to language processing mechanisms. Finally, I suggest that learning to orchestrate and capitalize on this atmosphere may help us to uncover and support untapped potential in those we serve.

In language intervention, our ultimate objective is natural and spontaneous use of language (remembering, in truth, that we usually settle for anything we can get). People want to *talk*. We certainly do not see the families of aphasic patients complaining, "My husband (or wife) just can't gesture any more!" Talking is the first thing people notice, expect, and desire. What this usually means is that "talking" is the first concern. The importance of comprehension is not only for itself. Rather, comprehension is a dire necessity underpinning the number one value—talking. Reading and writing skills are normally built on the foundation of speaking and listening competence. Whenever an individual shows potential for spoken language, reading and writing tend to become secondary communication channels.

Normally, spoken language appears and develops naturally and spontaneously. Research in the past decade has opened up vast, previously unexplored areas. These findings have illustrated the phonological, syntactic, semantic, and pragmatic patterning that underlies language use. We can now observe how patterns unfold in a developmental frame. These discoveries have resulted in a burst of clinical energy directed toward helping children and adults who have language difficulties. Assessment and remediation focus on these newly uncovered linguistic and pragmatic patterns. We do this because we know that such patterns are necessary for spontaneous language performance. However, we have paid scant attention to the special and unique character of spontaneous language and the ways in which spontaneous language using such patterns is generated. What is spontaneous language really like?

Spontaneous Language Is Not Consciously Generated

As with first steps taken by my daughter, most of the time we speak with very little conscious awareness of the specific patterns selected for use. Processing is not handled at the conscious level. Most of us know the intent of our utterances, but we must hear ourselves say something to know exactly how we have said it. For the most part, speech patterns are acquired and stored without our conscious awareness. Although talking is voluntary, speech once set in motion is highly automatic and is controlled at unconscious levels.

This idea is hardly novel. Few language researchers would dispute the statement that a child's language acquisition is accomplished without conscious attention to the processes that sort out sounds and their linguistic organizations. It could be argued that individuals in language training must learn by conscious effort to compensate for inadequately functioning processes at less conscious (i.e., subconscious or unconscious) levels. I return to this point later. Much of the language children and adults produce in the clinical setting is not truly spontaneous, because people have been made highly aware of what they are doing with their words. If language training is not spontaneous, does it engage the processes beneath our awareness that are the real determiners of most speech?

Some treatment approaches indirectly take this idea into account. For example, in the intensive stimulation approach to aphasia of Schuell, Jenkins, and Jiménez-Pabón (1964), the patient's dysfunctioning process system is stimulated through broad, yet intensive bombardment. The brain is left more or less on its own to assimilate what it finds useful. Martin (1978) has advocated a special type of conversational stimulation with unintelligible jargon patients. The clinician, after becoming familiar with an individual's error patterns and by controlling topic and context, begins to grasp and predict the speaking intent. This knowledge enables the clinician to respond meaningfully and opens the way for further communication. Over time, patients begin to use more and more of whichever processing maneuvers make it easier for the listener to grasp their intentions. Thus, intelligibility and form gradually increase. In this approach patients are not consciously aware of what they do that brings about improvement in communication. On the other hand, a patient's conscious awareness of improvement in communication may serve as a reinforcement for continued strategic attempts on levels that are not conscious.

Pinpointing the activation of linguistic processes beneath our awareness is not necessarily easy, as was brought to my attention during recent second-language research with children (Cochrane, 1980). The children were asked to discriminate and produce speech sounds at the syllable level. In pilot testing, the younger children (under 7 or 8 years) displayed difficulty in identifying which sound was different when they heard sample sounds they supposedly knew: [ba] — [da] — [da]. No child made errors on these sounds in his own speech, and all the children's imitations were entirely accurate. Clearly, at some undetermined, less conscious level they could differentiate /b/ from /d/ because their spontaneous speech demonstrated that ability. When given a specific identification task, they failed to make these distinctions. To conclude that children could not make these distinctions in language would be invalid. Often, we measure linguistic processes that normally occur without awareness by using testing procedures that involve the subject's awareness of purpose. Consequently, we may fail to engage speech processing mechanisms as they actually operate in ordinary language usage.

The question of which processes are engaged in the acquisition and use of speech can be equally unsettling in the language remediation context. For example, in aphasia diagnostics the preponderance of diagnostic information is not taken from a "spontaneous" speech sample, but from tasks involving a heightened awareness of required language performance. Such tests may be excellent for pinpointing isolated deficits, but they seem to be weak in measuring normal language use. Test information may not be particularly relevant to difficulties experienced in normal communication. Low test scores may seriously underrate communication ability and/or lead to the mistaken conclusion of poor learning potential. During testing, important linguistic processes go unrecognized and largely untested and, thus, untapped in treatment.

For example, individuals may fail a reading test at the single-word level but be able to get on the right bus that takes them to and from treatment. They may not be conscious of how they somehow decipher the bus sign. Often, patients are able to make social conversation although failing miserably on a naming task. One study of mentally retarded adults demonstrated that individuals whose test performance on certain syntactic structures was poor, could converse normally in certain conversational contexts (Bedrosian and Prutting, 1976).

Case of Mr. C.   In aphasia, the importance of language processing at the unconscious level was brought to my attention in an experience with a severely nonfluent patient. In working with Mr. C., data collection demonstrated that language retrieval could occur without the patient's conscious control and without improved performance in treatment or on standardized tests. Although after 6 months consistent improvement on a wide range of articulation had language tasks failed to be established in the clinic, the patient's wife reported that he occasionally produced a few clear words at home. Beginning at approximately 8 months after the cardiovascular accident (CVA) that had brought on the aphasia, Mrs. C. was able to record almost every understandable utterance over the subsequent 18-month period. The great majority of the patient's utterances remained unintelligible; however, development in both quality and quantity of intelligible output was clearly evidenced. These remarks could be documented in data from his spontaneous productions as seen in the samples displayed in Table 1. Table 2 indicates changes in output as measured by changes in the number and length of utterances over a 2-year period.

At this time I had found no technique I could use to support the recovery processes that seemed to be operating at some other level for this individual. Therefore, I was forced to conclude that the situations and contexts that stimulated his intelligible speech attempts had little relation to language stimulation tasks. This conclusion began my in-

Table 1.   Spontaneous utterances of Mr. C. sampled at about 8 months post-CVA and 18 month later

August 1977 (MLU 2.3)	March 1979 (MLU 5.2)
Don't go away.	I like to go out—too cold.
Honey.	No, I don't want anything.
Leave TV alone.	There it is again—thunder.
Billy, come back.	Did you pay him for it?
Do test.	What were you fixing for eat?
Grass.	See that boy up there?
Sit down.	Where we go for dinner?
Black clouds.	Leave car there, I walk.

Table 2.   Changes in output in mean length of utterance and use of
sentences for Mr. C. over a 2-year interval

Month	MLU	Number of sentences	Average sentences number/day
August 1977	2.3	42	1
November 1977	3.5	74	2
April 1978	5.2	104	3
September 1978	6.6	89	3
September 1979	4.6	214	7

ternal questioning of how to create a procedure for cooperating with
unconsciously operating linguistic processes already in operation.

Case of Mr. B.   In contrast, data collected on the spontaneous
output of another patient, Mr. B., seemed to demonstrate that intervention strategies showed potential for activating and promoting the
patient's spontaneous speech. During the first 5 months (January 1978
through May 1978; see Table 3) after his CVA, only minimal improvement in performance had been noticed. Then we began a new program
called "conversational prompting." Before this program, Mr. B. produced no spontaneous output outside treatment that could be charted.
As Tables 3 and 4 indicate, however, he showed steady progress in
mean length of utterance (MLU) and linguistic quality over the next 7
months in treatment.

The techniques used with this patient were unusual in what I now
regard are important ways. First, the clinician began by attempting to
create a realistic conversational atmosphere, using real objects, questions, and side remarks to maintain interest and flow. Second, many
clinical techniques were combined. Imitation abilities were fostered
through modeling, and multilevel cueing was used to elicit responses.
Through combinations of repetition and cue fading, while seeking to
maintain conversational openness and flow, I provided opportunities
to expand the structure of the intended utterance, and encouraged productions without cueing from me. During successive repetitions, cues

Table 3.   Changes in output in mean
length of utterance for Mr. B beginning
with the fifth month post-CVA

Month	MLU
January 1978	2.1
March 1978	3.2
May 1978	2.9
June 1978	4.6
November 1978	8.8

Table 4.   Examples of Mr. B's progress in sentence usage over 7 months of training

June 2, 1978 Total utterances = 18	February 15, 1979 Total utterances = 47
I am alone. I don't see that one. On the stomach. Put the plate on the table. Put the apple on the plate. Put the plate on the table right in front of the apple. Put the apple by the toothbrush. To/you are going to cut the cake. Which you're peeling.	I didn't have a heart attack. My brother-in-law had a heart attack and he died. Approximately a year ago. He had a heart attack before my time. He had a heart attack before I had my stroke. Yes, that is what I thought but he didn't make it. It was going on a long time. No, he lived in Houston.

were gradually reduced, then withheld altogether, as in the following example.

Clinician: *"Let's make a sandwich. Would you like one?"*
Mr. B.:   *"Yes."*
Clinician: *"Okay, tell me that. 'I would l_____.'"*
Mr. B.:   *"Like a sandwich."*
Clinician: *"Great! Ham or beef?"*
Mr. B.:   *"Ham."*
Clinician: *"See if you can tell me that. I would _____."*
Mr. B.:   *"Like a ham."*
Clinician: *"Ham — what?"*
Mr. B.:   *"Sandwich."*
Clinician: *"OK — Are you sure that's what you want? I don't like ham. But you do, huh?"*
Mr. B.:   *"Yes."*
Clinician: "OK — Tell me the whole thing."
Mr. B.:   *"I want —"*
Clinician: *"A h_____."*
Mr. B.:   *"A ham sandwich."*
Clinician: *"Fine. Now try to tell me the whole thing without help."*
Mr. B.:   *"I want a ham sandwich."*

   The data collected from speech used outside the clinic suggested that the treatment techniques might be tapping mechanisms underlying ordinary spontaneous speech production. Although much of the client's output during training seemed to be imitatively tied to the clinician input, and the language of the clinician often contained an artificial element of "reading into" patient intent, language used outside the clinic was not influenced by clinical technique. Later even this patient's speech in the clinic often surprised me in both form and content, as he used a high level of spontaneity along with his improved linguistic performance.

Gradually I was becoming aware that unexpected linguistic competence and, thus, potential for language retrieval could lie hidden and untouched, but might not be completely out of reach. Two other patients, both profoundly involved as measured by traditional testing, taught me not to underestimate linguistic competence or potential just because it was not demonstrable on conscious speaking and listening tasks.

Case of Mr. L.   No verbal program was attempted for the first 9 months of treatment because Mr. L. was stimulable for only three sounds. His partner in gestural treatment, however, had been able to use gestures as a speech facilitator and used gestures and speech together in treatment. Mr. L. did not enjoy being left out of speech attempts, so the clinician allowed him to try some short words that involved the three stimulable sounds. A few other sounds gradually became stimulable, using phonetic placement techniques. After several more months, he began to produce a few relevant single words (e.g., football, love, I). All productions were very distorted, slow, and painstaking, but were often identifiable. Although his test scores remained unchanged, at 14 months post-CVA he began to be stimulable for phrase completions and short sentences using the technique of conversational cueing described above. Many of his utterances contained appropriate, unmodeled syntactical forms and unexpected words from his own repertoire, as indicated:

(Context: a conversation about pets)

Clinician: *"Do you like to take your dog on walks?"*
Mr. L.:   (nods, yes)
Clinician: *"Tell me, you like to walk your dog."*
Mr. L.:   (smiles and says slowly and with distortion) *"AH — LAK — DOO — WAH — K — MAH — SHEP — UR — D."* [I like to walk my shepherd.]

Notice here that correct use of "I" and "my" indicates that Mr. L. was able to reformulate the model to fit his own intent. His [ʃ] was perfectly produced and had never been successfully stimulated, so it could not have been a conscious attempt. The clinician did not know he owned a shepherd, so the patient must be credited with a spontaneous production. Apparently he was using conscious techniques he learned in training for most sound productions. Yet, in producing words like "shepherd" without awareness, he was able to tap stored phonological and semantic material. Exactly what triggered his spontaneous mechanisms remains a mystery, but the important point is that until they were triggered, no one knew they were there, least of all the patient.

Case of Mr. M.   Another patient, Mr. M., displayed a similar test profile and laborious pattern of sound acquisition. Initially he did not respond to any verbal stimulation procedures for any sounds, though he seemed to be able to identify some short single words in written form. Like Mr. L., he was placed on a gesture program. Slowly, over 4 to 5 months, he began to produce distorted sounds in isolation. Here are some excerpts from a journal of his progress begun later, after about 20 sounds had been stimulated:

April 23   In conversational prompting, he cannot imitate the sound strings well enough, or transfer the production into the conversational context with enough consistency to make talking really successful. However, now he can imitate all the sounds on the drill chart in any order, if given as a separate task. With conversational prompting, some correct sounds will be emitted spontaneously. If I go back to the drill chart for needed sounds, he may often mispronounce them on the chart; he seems to perseverate on errors produced in the conversational context. He will often hear his errors and attempt correction, with inconsistent results.

May 8   Sometimes the conversational prompting works well. At other times he will try to put a string of sounds together and he's just miles off. I feel sure that his internal targets are correct. His failures must drive him crazy.

May 11   I started speeding up his sound drill to try to improve sound blending coordination.

June 1   I can't put my finger on what was amiss in this session. I believe he feels too much performance pressure from the look on his face when he misses target sounds in the conversation.

June 24   Mr. M. baffled me again, with a spontaneous production of the number "three" that was clear as a bell. Up to now it has always been a distorted combination of the drill sounds: /θ/ - /w/ - /ai/. I'm not sure how he accessed the word.

June 29   I'm getting some more nice improvement on numbers with Mr. M.

July 9   In conversational prompting, his rhythm on putting sounds together is improving, especially with written cues.

July 13   Today he said "two" as clear as a bell, although it's always been distorted. How is he accessing this?

July 15   I asked Mr. B. (Mr. M.'s treatment partner): "Tell me you'd like a trip to Florida," and Mr. M. popped up spontaneously with the whole sentence instead: "I want to go to Florida." (Florida mispronounced.) Notice: Mr. M. took the opportunity to speak when the pressure was on his *partner* to produce something. That was when he moved into the new level. Today he said "two" in his old, distorted way, and when I asked for a repeat, there it was again—perfect and clear, like before!

July 16   Mr. M. prompted into several short, semispontaneous sentences including: "I will take one bag." "Are you ready?" Who would have ever believed this man would produce sentences?

Case of Mr. D.   Data from these patients indicate undocumented language competence—processing abilities that remained after the injury and could be tapped through clinical interaction when phonological prerequisites were in place. The contrast between descriptions of conversation in the clinic and memorized speech patterns acquired in training was brought home unforgettably through work with another patient, Mr. D. He had acquired, as a result of extensive drill and a tremendous amount of perseverance, a limited number of consonants and vowels. I had tried to help him combine these in useful ways: "Hi," "Bye," "My way," "No," "I may," and so on. These words were finally drilled to the point of sounding fairly normal. The ones he did best on were "Hi," "Bye," and "No way!" When we caught sight of each other in the lobby, he stood up and smiled broadly. "Hi," I said. "No way!" he returned loudly and happily, entirely unaware of the inappropriateness of his response. I grieved inwardly over the long months of strenuous effort that were effectively nullified by this undesirable verbal example.

There is an old German legend about the owner of a vineyard. Because he complained so much, he was given a magic wand with power to control the weather. Happy at last, he watched the ground closely, and when it became dry he waved the wand and it would rain. Then the sun would shine again. Never had the vines produced such a beautiful crop. He could hardly wait to be the first to taste the grapes at harvest. To his dismay, they were so sour and bitter no one could eat them. The powers appeared, and taking his wand said, "You forgot the wind." Without pollenation the grapes had failed to sweeten. In programmed learning, as in the example of Mr. D., and his response "No way!" we successfully manipulate many variables, yet never seem to be able to control everything. On the other hand, the examples of Mr. B., Mr. L., and Mr. M., lead to a blending of traditional intervention strategies such as cueing and sound stimulation in an atmosphere designed to elicit responses that are less controlled, less conscious and, thus, more spontaneous.

Spontaneity in Speaking Decreases as Our Speech Awareness Increases

For a moment, picture yourself at a cocktail party. You are friendly and outgoing, but have met only a few of the guests previously. You smile and say hello, introducing yourself in order to start mingling. No one is particularly comfortable, and the talk centers on polite subjects—the weather, what occupations people have, and where they live. Then comes a gap in the conversation. You are casting about for something to say, trying out several topics and sentences in your mind, before speaking. When you finally say what you had planned, it sounds a little stiff. You are glad when food and drinks appear. Inhibitions begin to loosen, and your mood elevates with that of the group. Now you talk animatedly about something amusing that happened at work.

Effects of Environmental Demands   Tikofsky (1978) has pointed out that environmental demands create stress that in turn has important effects on language performance. Unfamiliar faces or situations, pressure to understand a fast flow of speech, and expectations for correct, nondelayed speech are stressful for us all, but are even more so for individuals with limitations in language processing capacities. Tikofsky stated that this extra burden negatively affects the brain's residual capacity and reduces our chances for maximizing potential. If this is true, language and remediation techniques that reduce rather than create such stress should be highly desirable. In addition to affecting consciousness about speech output, stress may also reduce language processing potential. Stress is not likely to have a positive influence on speech spontaneity, nor on its qualitative dimensions.

Usually, we're relieved and happy if we can begin to laugh and relax at a party. What is the function of light joking and laughter in this situation? Laughter is at once a response and a stimulus, an instant communicator of positive feelings. Because it is catching, laughter promotes nonverbal sharing and bonding between people. Also, laughter is usually relaxing. It is of particular interest to us that laughter promotes spontaneity. When laughter erupts, delight overcomes decorum and stiffness dissolves. Laughter can ease the anxiety and fear that often hinder spontaneity. We have all attended parties at which this process failed to occur, and the atmosphere never allowed an easy, natural, and spontaneous conversational flow.

Speech is usually a means to an end, and when excessive conscious attention is given to it, spontaneity suffers. When the atmosphere is unfamiliar, stiff, or forced, because everyone is trying too hard, spontaneity is like a cocktail party that never gets off the ground. This analysis holds interesting implications for language remediation techniques. Often language training, for both children and adults, is characterized by "pumping." Pumping is what clinicians learn to do to create opportunities for targeted verbal responses. It works like artificial respiration. The clinician attempts to stimulate the client's language system by forcing it into operation. Techniques used are repeats ("Say it again"), imitations ("Say 'I want the ball'"), indirect commands ("Tell me you want the ball"), questions ("Where shall I throw it?"), paraphrases ("Did you say throw it or kick it?"), sentence completions ("Throw the _____"), memorized answers (Stimulus: "What do you say?" Response: "Throw the ball."), and many other clever maneuvers. In discussing "forced responses" and their artificiality in language production, Winitz (1981) has emphasized the importance of meaningfulness and comprehensibility in normal language acquisition, and how normal language acquisition is devoid of drill forms.

Language associated with pumping frequently lacks spontaneity. Spontaneity can be blocked in at least three ways. First, when speech and language are created primarily by the clinician, spontaneity is given to the clinician and taken away from the client. Second, when clinical tasks draw attention to speech output, the resulting increase in speech awareness will curtail speech spontaneity. The alternative is to create tasks that can function so that speech output is a by-product of the situation, analogous to the effect the appearance of the dog had for my 12-month-old daughter. Tasks that focus minimally on linguistic performance and contain some other objective can often create language in the process. Here the language user is not self-conscious about the use of language that results when attention is given to language tasks. The clinical task can encourage active awareness, but at the same time attention is focused away from spontaneous speech output so that internal language mechanisms can operate more naturally. Thus, spontaneity in the use of language is subtly encouraged. The third block to spontaneity involves the loss of the openness and flow that occurs in normal conversations, yet is often difficult to maintain in the clinical setting. The stronger the orientation to accomplish a certain task, the more the task can get in the way of conversational flow, actually blocking language spontaneity. The clinician can ease this difficulty by attention to the communicative interplay between persons, instead of emphasizing the completion of a task or the correction of an error. In this approach, planning is important, for without a plan conversational energies will not be initiated. And yet, the plan cannot be allowed to overwhelm the conversational flow it creates.

Using Communicative Interplay   Two recent aphasia group activities that were successful in this regard illustrate how this interplay can work. In the first instance, the task was initiated by creating a group "fantasy vacation trip," which ended up in a country chosen by the group. In this introduction, the clinician simply asked leading questions, encouraged group responses through questions, (e.g., "Where shall we go first?" "How will we get to Canada?" "How long shall we stay?"), guided the group to achieve consensus, and attempted to get it to verbalize the plan. Then the clinician announced that in Albania (the final country in the plan that evolved), the group would meet an expert who would teach about Albanian customs. The second clinician then donned a funny hat, and looking important said he was the Albanian expert and would show the group how to make an Albanian place setting for a meal. He read a list of humorous and unlikely instructions (e.g., "Put the knife in the glass."). The clinician's role was to manipulate various objects set up on the table. However, the clinician purposely made errors in following the instructions. The group's task was to make sure the instructions were followed to the letter. Group members delighted in telling the clinician about her mistakes, and they even interrupted each other in their eagerness to speak. After being corrected by a group member, the clinician innocently continued to move something the wrong way—"Oh, to the left of the plate? Okay" (moving it to the right instead). Some patients were so involved that they stood up or rolled their wheelchairs over to the table, grabbing items to put them in the correct place. The clinician used this as a further opportunity, laughing and saying, "Oh! I see. Now, what did you just do?"

In another group activity, the original task as planned was to pass out colored felt pieces in preparation for a game. However, the "passing out" phase turned out to be so rich in conversational opportunity that the game was never played. Instead, the clinician guided the situational responses. For example, three patients agreed that they would like a blue piece, so the clinician asked the group who should have it and people responded with their own opinions and rationales. The clinician gave patients colors other than those they had asked for, which prompted laughter and requests for changes. The clinician gave some patients more pieces than others and then asked, "Who needs another one?" Then the group members began noticing and counting each other's pieces. One patient got carried away. Standing up and pointing, he exclaimed, "He's got one, he's got three, he's got two, I got two. There's three of them right there. He's got two over there, and he's only got one." Then his neighbor on the right finished it off: "And one over here."

This task has been described not only to demonstrate that the apparent task may differ from the real conversational objective; it also indicates how a simple task can generate a good conversational flow. Such a task can easily deteriorate into a pumping technique, however:

clarity of purpose is essential. From this standpoint many traditional language tasks can be used to generate conversational flow. Reemphasis is needed so that the objective of spontaneous communication can be realized. It may be possible to transform the role of the clinician from "pumping" speech output to promoting tasks to generate spontaneous flow, to guiding the flow of conversation by focusing on the flow as the basic objective.

To encourage spontaneity of language, we should consider ways to move away from conscious, effortful speech attempts. Conscious, effortful speech may not only fail to engage our normal internal processing mechanisms, but may actively interfere with the expression of spontaneous language.

Spontaneous Language Fits the Person

Unlike my daughter, another child watching the entry of a dog into the yard might have chosen to ignore him, or might have shown some other response, such as fear or curiosity. Motivation for expression comes from within, whether its purpose is derived externally or internally. Compare the variety of styles and intents found in these examples:

Mr. C.:   *"There it is again . . . thunder."*
   A person who loved nature, weather, and anything outside
Mr. B.:   *"Approximately a year ago."*
   An intellectual rancher
Mr. S.:   *"There's three of them right there."*
   A construction worker.

There are many possible ways to express an idea, but the expression *fits* the person that produces it. An individual's own cognitive frame, imagination, reaction potential, personality style, and motives all influence the content of spontaneous utterances.

As previously noted, the "pumping" technique may constrain spontaneity by undue attention to a person's speech. If in "pumping" we place preconceived expectations on the situation and its speech outcomes, we may also unwittingly thwart spontaneity by discouraging individual expression, which is the freedom to respond in a manner corresponding to personal style, desires, purposes, needs, history, expectations, and abilities. When specific behaviors are necessary, such as in teaching fire drill procedures, a directive approach is justified. In allowing children to develop their own procedures for getting out of a school building in case of fire, a principal invites disaster. But where spontaneity is constrained by prescriptive teaching of certain forms or responses, individual and personal factors cannot be used to promote self-expression.

Yet, at times, clinicians need to attend to situations in which the child or adult repeatedly avoids the use of certain language forms or uses deviant language. What method can be used that does not violate spontaneity? One possibility is to use feedback to guide spontaneous responses into forms that will communicate more effectively. Repetition, modeling, corrective feedback, and other techniques are useful as long as we do not lose sight of this goal.

The closer the patient's output comes to being spontaneous, the closer we come to realizing our fundamental treatment objectives. As long as we recognize where we wish to go, through emphasis on spontaneous use, we can accept and support communication through intermediary steps as needed. However, we must learn to use clinical techniques in ways that do not impede spontaneity.

Spontaneous Speech Is Wedded to Its Context

In some sense separation of speech output from its context is futile. Spontaneous speech arises from within a broader, contextual experience. This larger experience includes an environmental setting containing a great deal of peripheral information. The setting is grasped in relation to past perceptions and experience, but the experience exists only for its particular moment.

What does this consideration tell us about the quality of clinical language experiences? Examine the following clinical interactions for their power to engage spontaneous conversational flow:

1. Clinician (showing picture of gas station): *"What is this?"*
    Response: *"Gas station."*
2. Clinician (showing a picture of a man in a car at a filling station): *"What is going on here?"*
    Response: *"He wants some gas."*
    Clinician: *"Does he want anything else?"*
    Response: *"I don't know."*
3. Clinician (showing same picture): *"What would this man in the picture say?"*
    Response: *"Fill it up."*
    Clinician: *"Anything else?"*
    Response: *"Check the oil."*
4. Clinician: *"Let's imagine you're driving in your car, and you glance at the gas gauge—oh oh, what might be wrong?"*
    Response: *"I'm low on gas."*
    Clinician: *"What will you do?"*
    Response: *"Go and get some."*

Clinician: *"Is there a station close by?"*
Response: *"No, about 2 miles away."*
Clinician: *"OK, suppose we go there. I'll be the attendant and you tell me what you want. Hello, sir, what will you have?"*
Response: *"Fill it up."*
Clinician: *"Regular, lead free, or super?"*
Response: *"Lead free."*
Clinician: *"Sorry, sir, we just ran out of lead free."*
Response: *"My car won't run on anything else."*

In the first two examples, context is provided by a picture and the patient's speech is limited to a description of it. In the third example, the context is again provided, but the client is asked to project an appropriate, imaginary verbalization.

What makes the last example seem more real and spontaneous than the others? Here, image building creates an immediate, personal context within which the two conversational interactions are generated. Although speech is practiced, the initial interplay helps build the context for the experiential reality in role playing. Importantly, the client becomes a part of the action. Spontaneous, imaginary, and even unexpected variables are allowed to shape the experience. Thus, stimulation becomes more realistic as responses are tied to the actual moment. The experience is richer than the pictured context, and the client is encouraged to help create and respond to a reality containing immediate demands and opportunities. The output cannot be entirely predicted until it occurs.

Normally, speech is acquired as one aspect of our larger, contectual experience, whereas isolating speech from its context deprives it of its essential relations. Because of this isolation, much of our language remediation is analogous to learning to ride a bicycle by sitting in midair turning the pedals round and round—there is no street, no turning or braking decisions to be made, no steering or balancing needed, no destination built into this exercise. Is it any wonder transfer of this beautifully learned pedaling behavior to real bicycling may prove difficult? Spontaneous speech is real speech, operating in relation to all the factors that engender, affect, and react to it. In treatment, the closer we can come to creating a rich experiential reality, the more speech shares in that reality.

Our concern is beyond that of making the language of treatment pragmatically useful. Language must be integrated with the larger set of nonverbal communication behaviors such as eye contact, gestures, emotional tone, and body language, as well as the social and psychological environment in which the communication occurs.

CONCLUSIONS

We have explored several dimensions of spontaneous language. We have observed that because spontaneous language is not generated at a conscious level, we need to seek new ways of discovering and tapping its potential. In addition, we have observed that conscious attention to speech production can be counterproductive to speech spontaneity. Also, I have stressed the personal character of speech, along with the inseparability of spontaneous language from the experiences that generate it.

The factors I have described are not new. But to acknowledge their vital importance in both language acquisition and retrieval, and to seek to make more use of them, is new. My purpose here is not to detail all the steps in an adventurous clinical approach. It *is* of primary importance that spontaneity and unconscious processes form our overall objective and that our challenge is to begin creating clinical instruments geared to this level of interaction and intervention. To seek a new direction is enough at this moment. Once we have sensed our destination, we can attend fully to the steps that will take us forward.

We now need to concentrate on a new direction, a conscious clinical strategy designed to motivate and sustain a level of spontaneous participation that I have termed "the atmosphere of delight." I have chosen the word "delight" with a definite purpose. The idea of "delight" reaches beyond the objective of creating interesting learning tasks into an area not previously considered. When delight has entered our treatment process, it has been the result of the personality of a clinician or client rather than an aspect of treatment that could be approached deliberately and purposefully.

As in the case of my daughter's first steps, we could observe delight functioning and sense its power, yet why or how it worked was not explained. In working with aphasia, I have observed moments when its importance seemed obvious. Such results have been rewarding and have led me to propose that we begin systematically to create clinical tasks and environments where spontaneity and delight can become central facilitators for the learning and retrieval process.

Imagine delight appearing on the face of someone you know. Whether delight is imagined, observed, or expressed, it is a positive, pleasurable experience. Delight is associated with intrinsic interest, with fun, with ease, with enjoyment. Above all delight is spontaneous—it suggests a pleasant surprise. An atmosphere containing delight is inviting, like the feeling at a good party. Thus, our clinical objective would be to create and sustain an atmosphere containing fun, surprise, interest, ease, invitation, laughter, and spontaneity. What is the purpose of this atmosphere for us? Chiefly, to utilize the characteristics of comfortable, pleasurable experiences to further spontaneous interaction in the clinical setting. Tedious or difficult work stimulates delight in practically no one. In contrast, evoking an atmosphere of delight serves us in numerous ways.

Language tasks that are structured for the purpose of creating and maintaining a climate of delight and interest will encourage spontaneous involvement and self-expression. Practice takes place within a safe, positive, yet real communication experience. As speech anxiety and speech demands are reduced, laughter, relaxation, interest, and delight can take their place. The clinical atmosphere, like a good party, is created to warm the participants, to reduce their inhibitions, and to involve them more and more in ongoing activity.

Laughter as a manifestation of delight becomes a clinical instrument that is associated with relaxation, spontaneous interactions, and sharing. In turn, each of these promotes spontaneous language attempts, meaning that language processing will occur at less conscious levels. Laughter can also be a useful tool in providing a positive alternative to failure. In an atmosphere of delight, failure can be transformed because all attempts to communicate can receive recognition and support.

The purpose of delight is to provide an atmosphere that evokes real, spontaneous communication among participants. It involves creating a clinical style in keeping with the atmosphere. The clinician becomes a vehicle of communication, acting as a guide to the flow of conversation, action, and energy, as well as an intervention strategist. Critical feedback and pressure through "pumping" are avoided because they induce self-awareness, stress, and anxiety.

A teaching approach that emphasizes the importance of atmosphere in the learning situation has been used successfully in second language learning and in teaching academic subjects to elementary school children (Lozanov, 1979). The strength of this approach is that spontaneous communication taps into the processing mechanisms used in real communication, but often left untouched in language. However, if clients were made aware of the purposes, objectives, and intervention techniques being used in this approach, they could participate at two levels: by responding to the clinician's intent, and, at the same time, doing it spontaneously.

In this way, clinician and client could share the responsibility for the learning process, and, in turn, enable all processes to serve overall communication development. Guided by the atmosphere of delight, perhaps language potential will begin to show its true face, and a natural and effective communication approach will evolve.

REFERENCES

Bedrosian, J., and Prutting, C. 1976. The communicative performance of the mentally retarded adult in four conversational settings. Unpublished paper.

Cochrane, R. M. 1980. The acquisition of R and L by Japanese children and adults learning English as a second language. J. Multilingual Multicultural Dev. 1(4):331–360.

Lozanov, G. 1979. Suggestology and Outlines of Suggestopedy. Gordon & Breach, New York.

Martin, A. D. 1978. Therapeutic intervention with the fluent aphasic. Paper presented at the American Speech, Language and Hearing Association Convention, Chicago, 1978.

Schuell, H., Jenkins, J. J., and Jiménez-Pabón, E. 1964. Aphasia in Adults: Diagnosis, Prognosis, and Treatment. Hoeber, New York.

Tikofsky, R. S. 1978. Aphasia: A problem of sociolinguistic information processing. Commun. Disord. Audio J. Contin. Educ. 3(2).

Winitz, H. 1981. Linear and nonlinear learning. In: H. Winitz (ed.), The Comprehension Approach to Foreign Language Instruction. Newbury House, Rowley, Mass.

CHAPTER 10

Communication Styles of Fluent Aphasic Clients

Robert C. Marshall

> *Marshall illustrates the communication styles of fluent aphasics. He addresses the difficulty they have in communication and outlines treatment procedures.*
>
> 1. *Marshall summarizes recent approaches to the treatment of aphasia. Do you understand the following approaches: cueing, Melodic Intonation Therapy, and deblocking? (See Chapter 11 for a complete description of deblocking.)*
> 2. *What is Marshall's position on the value of classification systems for aphasic clients? What type of classification system is he referring to? Do you agree? How does the author define fluent aphasia?*
> 3. *In talking about the communication styles of fluent aphasic patients, Marshall indicates five serious problem areas. What are they? Discuss each one and contrast it with the others.*

WITHIN THE PAST 15 YEARS, significant evidence has accumulated to indicate that speech and language rehabilitation enhances recovery from aphasia beyond the point of spontaneous resolution (Basso, Capitani, and Vignolo, 1979; Broida, 1977; Hagen, 1973; Holland, 1980b; Marshall, Tompkins, and Phillips, 1982; Sarno and Levita, 1979; Wertz et al., 1982). Although these investigations have stimulated favorable comments on aphasia rehabilitation (Benson, 1979), it is often difficult, because of the methodological constraints of group design, to ascertain the effects of treatment for individual clients. Fortunately, the benefits of speech and language training have also been demonstrated with aphasic individuals who differ in type and severity of aphasia (Helm and Barresi, 1980; Kushner and Winitz, 1977; Simmons and Zorthian, 1979). It is important to recognize, however, that the criterion measure for change in many group and individual studies is performance on a standardized test, which may or may not have relevance to how the client communicates under normal circumstances. This underscores the importance of treatment for the individual and suggests that specific measures on tests or tasks (e.g., naming, comprehension, writing) are somewhat limited when communication for daily living is considered.

The central issue today is not whether aphasia treatment "works" but what kind of treatment works and with whom. This question, succinctly summarized in 1977 in an editorial in the Lancet, has been the subject of two large Veterans Administration Cooperative Studies. In addition, the past two decades have seen the development of a number of treatments designed to improve the speech and language production of particular types of aphasic disorders. Paramount among these efforts have been techniques to facilitate word retrieval (Love and Webb, 1977; Marshall, 1976), procedures to improve syntactic usage (Beyn and Shokhor-Trotskaya, 1966; Helm-Estabrooks, Fitzpatrick, and Barresi, 1981; Naeser, 1975), and those designed to increase the verbalization of aphasic clients with limited verbal output. Among the techniques employed to increase clients' verbalization are innovations such as deblocking (Rosenbek, Collins, and Wertz, 1976), Melodic Intonation Therapy (Sparks, Helm, and Albert, 1974), and various other programs for improving the verbal productions of apraxic and apraxic–aphasic clients (Rosenbek et al., 1973; Dabul and Bollier, 1976; Deal and Florance, 1978).

Both external and internal cueing techniques are used to facilitate word retrieval by aphasic persons. In external cueing the clinician provides a stimulus to trigger production of a desired response. For example, if the target utterance is the word "pie," the clinician may use the carrier phrase, "I'd like a piece of apple _____" to elicit the word from the client. Internal cues are spontaneously produced by aphasic persons as they attempt to retrieve specific words in conversation and naming. For example, an aphasic individual might say "Oh it's good, you know, apple, pumpkin, berry, I love it," when trying to retrieve the word "pie." Accordingly, the clinician might ask the client to attend to these internal cues, if he or she feels it will facilitate production of the desired word.

Many aphasic persons communicate exclusively in the present tense. Others omit the function words of speech or employ what has been termed "telegraphic speech." For example, the client may say "Go beach Sunday," for "I am going to the beach on Sunday." Various instructional procedures have been employed to expand and enrich the syntactic structure used by aphasic persons. One excellent example is that provided by Helm-Estabrooks et al. (1981), who designed a syntax stimulation program using a hierarchy of eight sentence constructions to increase the phrase length and use of grammatical constructions of clients with Broca's aphasia.

Melodic Intonation Therapy (MIT) is a technique developed for severely nonfluent aphasics who demonstrate extreme paucity of speech and concern for their incapacity to communicate. MIT is a hierarchically presented program based on singing. It involves the use of intoned utterances, melody patterns, and rhythm, and relies heavily on clinician modeling and client repetition.

The technique of deblocking involves the stimulation of an intact communicative channel to facilitate ultimately the use of the severely impaired channel. In this vein, aphasic clients with marked deficits in verbal communication have been encouraged to use gestural or graphic modalities (intact channels) to deblock the impaired verbal channel.

Apraxia of speech, which frequently co-occurs with aphasia, is an articulatory disorder resulting from a brain injury that results in an impairment of the capacity to order the positioning of speech musculature and to sequence muscle movements for production of phonemes and phoneme sequences. Treatment of the disorder concentrates on the disordered articulation; it involves drills, repetition, teaching, and compensatory strategies and usually follows a specified hierarchy.

As indicated above, the client who is markedly limited in verbal skills or is nonfluent can be treated with a variety of techniques aimed at increasing or improving verbal output. Conspicuously lacking in the literature of aphasia, however, are accounts of treatment efficacy and procedures for clients who have little difficulty with verbalization, specifically, fluent aphasias. Aside from the efforts of Martin (1981), Whitney (1975), and the communication centered approaches stimulated by recent interest in language pragmatics (Davis and Wilcox, 1981; Holland, 1977; Wepman, 1972), the management of fluent clients has received little consideration.

The disproportionate number of treatment techniques available to clinicians for use with nonfluent patients stems from several factors. To begin with, there seem to be many more nonfluent than fluent aphasic patients. Studies by Benson (1967) and more recently by Kertesz and McCabe (1977) indicate that fluent patients usually have a lesion posterior to the Rolandic fissure sparing the motor strip. Consequently, they exhibit little physical impairment, require limited hospitalization, and most likely are seen by the speech-language pathologist as outpatients. In some instances, they escape the attention of the speech-language pathologist entirely or are discharged without being referred for evaluation. The disordered, fluent speech exhibited by these patients can sometimes be the only residual of neurologic insult. Finally, it is easy to design and to implement management procedures for nonfluent patients. Their limited output places control of the interaction in the hands of the clinician, who can determine with a prompt, a cue, or a question when and what the client will say; limited output, furthermore, simplifies the assessment and recording of the client's responses. Such precision and control are not easily achieved in management of the fluent client.

CLASSIFICATION OF APHASIC CLIENTS

According to Goodglass and Kaplan (1972), and central to the "Boston School of aphasia" are the premises that various components of the language system may be selectively affected by brain damage and that the impairment and/or preservation of specific language functions (e.g., repetition, fluency, comprehension) after brain injury provides a clue to anatomical organization of language in the brain and to the location of the lesion. The individual with Wernicke's aphasia, for example, incurs damage to Wernicke's area, which involves the posterior portion of the first temporal gyrus of the dominant hemisphere (usually the left). The speech and language features of diagnostic value for these clients include impaired auditory comprehension and fluently articulated paraphasic speech. The causative lesion for the conduction aphasic patient is usually deep to the supramarginal gyrus of the left cerebral hemisphere; it interrupts the arcuate fasciculus, a tract of fibers connecting Wernicke's area (temporal lobe) and Broca's area (frontal lobe). Primary symptoms that suggest a diagnosis of conduction aphasia involve disproportionate impairment in repetition skill in the presence of near-normal auditory comprehension.

Not surprisingly, the classification of aphasic syndromes has prompted many collaborative investigations among neurobehavioral scientists. These efforts add to our knowledge of aphasia and yield insights into the mysteries of the brain itself. Their contribution to and role in the rehabilitation of the aphasic person, however, is questionable. My purpose here, however, is not to revise aphasia classification systems, nor to minimize the diagnostic value of this process. Classification efforts show no signs of abating and reflect the ever-increasing vitality of a number of interrelated disciplines for which there is interest in the problems of aphasic persons. Nevertheless it is the clinician who is responsible for maximizing and/or improving the aphasic client's ability to communicate in society. And most clinicians who assume this responsibility would argue that it is sometimes difficult to classify reliably aphasic syndromes. Goodglass (1981) has suggested that "fewer than half of the patients with aphasia can be assigned with confidence to one of the standard syndromes." Kertesz and McCabe (1977) and others (Wertz, Kitselman, and Deal, 1981) have shown that aphasic clients move from one category to another in the recovery process. Thus it may be helpful to consider some new strategies in planning treatment for aphasic individuals in addition to those based on classification schema.

This chapter approaches treatment of selected fluent aphasic clients through analysis of their communication styles in communicative interactions. "Management," as used in this chapter, means modification, augmentation, or alteration of the client's communication style to maximize information exchange during interactions. The point of view represented in this chapter is similar to that taken in mental health management in which the need to classify (e.g., as schizophrenic, manic-depressive, etc.) is of secondary importance to modification and/or elimination of the behaviors that contribute to the individual's maladaptive functioning in society.

FEATURES OF COMMUNICATION STYLE

"Communication style" refers to the manner in which the aphasic person transmits and receives information in natural communicative interactions. Natural interactions are events in which clients participate in conducting their daily activities. For example, the following interaction took place between a 67-year-old fluent aphasic man and a store clerk:

Aphasic man: *"I'd like one of those."* (points to cigarettes)
Clerk: *"A pack of Winstons?"* (reaches for Winstons)

Aphasic man: *"No, one more this way."* (points to right of Winstons)
Clerk: *"Oh!, You mean the Kools?"*
Aphasic man: *"That's the one. The big ones.*
Clerk: *"The king size. OK, here you are."*
Aphasic man: (counting change) *"Here's some stuff."*
Clerk: *"That stuff I need. Thank you."*

The exchange provides an example of an aphasic person making a request without using any specific words. It also highlights a major thrust in aphasia treatment today, namely, it is how the individuals communicate (successfully or unsuccessfully), not whether they say the correct words, that really matters in getting along in life. This ability seems to be particularly important for fluent aphasic persons, and this chapter examines some of the communication styles used by these patients in situations similar to the one just illustrated.

No doubt several elements contribute to an individual's communication style. We can all recall patients who, in spite of many negative factors, were adept at keeping communication flowing; others, with standardized test results reflecting glowing potential, were inept at carrying out basic communications. Our patients, like our peers, use styles that stimulate or inhibit interaction. Elements that have potential for determining the communication style of the aphasic client include premorbid personality (introversion-passive vs. extroversion-active), need for verbal communication, capacity to cope with adversity (e.g., a stroke), and severity and type of aphasia. The interactions among these elements, and others not yet known, determine the communication style used by patients as they recover from and adjust to their permanent neurologic residuals.

This chapter describes three fluent aphasic communication styles and suggests some techniques to augment and modify these styles to enhance information exchange. Initially, however, we discuss some of the behavioral attributes that provide the theoretical basis for communication style analyses.

Comprehension

Communication is an interactive process with each participant serving as speaker (sender) and listener (receiver). Comprehension does not refer to auditory comprehension ability only, but to the general processes involved in an individual's willingness to verify and to seek clarification of information. Comprehension involves active listening, which includes attention to nonverbal messages supplied by the other participant in the interaction (facial expressions and other signs that indicate boredom). The client with a high sense of concern for comprehension actively listens by seeking verification through repetition and explanation. Because of their high concern for comprehension, these individuals may even ask their listeners to verify that they have understood. Conversely, individuals with limited concern for comprehension are reluctant to accept or take the role of receiver; rather, they press on incessantly with their own verbalizations. If they are forced to listen, they may tune out and simply wait to begin talking again.

Self-Monitoring

Aphasic individuals vary markedly in awareness of language production errors and in their ability to correct these errors (Marshall and Tompkins, 1982; Wepman, 1958). Martin (1981), in his comments on the treatment of jargon aphasia, spoke of intrapersonal and interpersonal monitoring. Intrapersonal monitoring refers to the process of self-correction and involves attention to language structure and usage, such as the selection of a phoneme or word, the determination of word order, and the preference for a particular phrase. Interpersonal monitoring refers to the act of attending to signals from the environment and from the other participant in the interaction that are important for sustaining communication; these signals indicate when it is appropriate to change roles or observe social convention (e.g., be quiet, don't smoke, wait in line).

Intrapersonal monitoring can facilitate communication if carried out with some degree of propriety. Excessive correction, however, may interfere with information exchange. Simply stated, there is a point at which enough "stabs" have been made at a word, and communication becomes secondary to production. No doubt there is an opportune time for each individual to accept an approximation or related substitution that communicates the intent of the message and maintains the interaction. Some aphasic clients realize this; others continue to correct and recorrect until the thought has been lost and both speaker and listener become frustrated. Aphasic clients who respond well to interpersonal cues may get along well in life, regardless of the severity of their language deficit. Others, however, remain oblivious to situations demanding social conformity or to signals that their messages are not being received. I recall a patient who was so impaired in interpersonal monitoring after a stroke that rendered him a fluent aphasic that he was taken by the police to a mental institution. That this happened immediately after the insult was not surprising because the stroke had occurred in a tavern. What did amaze me, however, was that despite his efforts to convey his language problem, the man spent 3 months in the institution before anyone discovered that he had a language disorder.

Awareness of Content

External cues of sentence completion ("You eat soup with a _____"), semantic association ("knife, fork, and _____"), initial phonemes (sp_____), oral spelling, or rhyme ("Not a moon but a _____") may all be useful in prompting specific words from nonfluent clients. Except for mildly dysnomic patients, however, fluent aphasic persons are not very responsive to these cues. Yet many individuals emit specific content words in their conversational discourse. The realization that specific content words have been produced varies from patient to patient. Some reflect this awareness with statements such as "Well, I said it that time but I can't all the time." Others do not seem to notice the content words they produce, but fixate on the words they cannot produce. Patients who are aware that they have produced a desired word are able to keep a conversation moving; those who do not notice "how well they have really done" tend to repeat themselves, and perseverate on similar themes throughout the interaction.

Self-Criticism

The fluent paraphasic utterances of some aphasic speakers are sometimes bizarre. An elderly client once asked me (with much concern) "How can it be that my kitchenships are placed before my substance had been pastured completely?" It is difficult to understand how patients fail to notice the bizarreness of such utterances. Yet there are some individuals who are completely unaware of their faulty communication, a condition described as "anosognosia for speech" (Kertesz, 1979). At the other extreme are the clients who are so acutely aware of their deficits that they constantly interrupt and disrupt their communications with self-critical statements such as "I'm crazy" and "I'm stupid," or apologize unnecessarily. This behavior, in my opinion, is unrelated to the severity of the deficit. There are individuals who are superb communicators yet spend much time demeaning themselves.

Compensatory Efforts

Compensatory efforts refer to word retrieval efforts that facilitate communication when there is no external prompting. Some individuals gesture, draw, write, spell, orally explain, describe, or show the listener what they want. Some compensate by attempting to cue the listener that they are "close" to conveying their message. For example, one patient trying to say the word "matches" produced a series of approximations ("batches, hatches, patches") and stated, "That's almost it, but not quite." Another interesting compensatory behavior is that of getting the listener to produce the desired word. For example, the patient may say "You know, the place where I was before I came here" (his home) or "the one I've been with for years and years" (his wife) and stimulate the listener to fill in the blanks. Some clients show excellent compensatory skills, but others talk on, and place all the burden on the listener to figure out what is being said.

COMMUNICATION STYLES: MANAGEMENT

The next sections describe three communication styles that I frequently see and offer suggestions for modifying these styles to improve communication. I consider only interactions that are natural, verbal, and involve two or more persons, one being the aphasic client.

Style 1: The Rambler

The term "rambler" describes fluent patients who dominate communicative interactions with their verbosity. These individuals are described as manifesting "logorrhea" in the French literature (Lecours et al., 1981) and with far less esoteric terms by their wives and contemporaries. Typically, ramblers demonstrate low interest in comprehension because they seem not to listen and/or to listen with difficulty. The self-correctional skills of ramblers are variable. Some are skilled in intrapersonal monitoring and are able to correct and revise production errors. Clients who are keenly aware of the content elements in their speech are especially skilled in this regard. Such patients are not difficult to understand; at times they are interesting conversationalists, but ultimately, their incessant verbalization wears on the listener. For ramblers who are poor in intrapersonal monitoring and unaware of their speech content, the listener experiences a different problem. The speech of these patients is highly paraphasic; it is difficult to transcribe, and it makes no sense. Although these patients may attract strange glances, they talk on and on, expecting, sometimes demanding, that their listeners understand what they are saying. Unfortunately, after a few seconds of listening to such a patient, most people are hopelessly lost.

It is in the interpersonal ability to monitor that ramblers truly have difficulties. They are usually so concerned with domination of the conversation that they fail to pick up information from the environment. They seem to be unaware of how much they talk. The treatment session for such a patient usually ends because of clinician fatigue rather than on an agreed on schedule. The compensatory skills of the rambler are also typically poor. Their major efforts in this area are verbal: explanation, description, circumlocution. These efforts may become so elaborate that meaning is lost. The use of gestures, showing the listener what is meant, or writing, usually forces ramblers to stop talking and provides opportunities for the listeners to speak. These helpful compensatory techniques are not used or tolerated by ramblers.

Treatment With ramblers, it is important that the clinician achieve some control of the interaction. Because ramblers are intense in their desire to dominate the conversation, the clinician may need to match this intensity to halt the one-way conversational flow. It is helpful to use exaggerated gestures and strong statements of agreement followed by a statement that the client must attend to keep the interaction going. For example, a very intense rambler was filibustering on how long it was taking a crew of painters to finish work on an outside wall of the hospital. After he had ranted and raved for several minutes, the clinician abruptly threw up his hands and exclaimed with equal irritation, "Oh my gosh, you are right; it is impossible to get good work any more. Let me tell you about what happened at my house." The client was placed in the position of having to listen for a few seconds, and a one-way conversation was recast into a two-way interaction.

It is easy to be mesmerized by the speech of the rambling patient we understand or to tune out the individual who loses us quickly in a cacophony of jargon. The clinician must be alert, however, for opportunities to effect a role switch. This may be done by using understanding statements such as "I see what you mean," by paraphrasing what the patient has said, or by requesting clarification. It is not that the client is unable to observe the rules of conversational turn taking. If the speech flow of the rambler can be reduced, a change can be made. When this has been accomplished, the clinician must quickly determine whether the topic of conversation should be continued, expanded, or changed.

When asking the rambler a question, carefully phrase it so that a short answer is the only way a patient can respond. Forced choices (e.g. "I understand you're going home this weekend. Is it Saturday or Sunday?") or yes/no questions (Is it raining now?) are the easiest means to elicit short answers. This approach tends to limit the opportunity for the rambler to respond with lengthy verbal statements and to promote turn taking.

When all else fails, honesty may be the best policy. Because of his hyperverbal behavior, the rambler may find that except for the clinician, few people will listen to him. Normal listeners, unlike the clinician who is attentive and empathetic, can display signs of lack of interest when listening becomes unpleasant. Ramblers who find themselves in this position may depend on the clinician, who may choose to exploit this relationship and request that the rambler stop talking and start listening when the occasion warrants. The tactfulness with which the aforementioned request must be made cannot be overstated.

Style 2: The Monitor

The hallmark of the monitor is an overabundance of self-correction. Monitors spend so much time correcting and revising production errors that their thoughts are not always followed or become lost in the process of correction. With this tendency to overcorrect, the monitor seems to show a high awareness of speech content. This awareness is, however, overshadowed by concern for production. Some patients are intolerant of their approximations, or their correction efforts lead them even farther from the intended target. If they do produce the target utterance, they may try to repeat it several times "to make it stick," but each time end up with an even poorer result.

These patients exhibit adequate concern for comprehension. Moreover, monitors are keenly aware of their verbal deficits. This may be displayed with temper outbursts or statements such as "Why can't I say that word?" Monitors are also very insistent on letting you know that they can say a word, that the word is "easy" or is on the tip of their tongue. Sometimes they blame their production problems on unrelated factors such as poorly fitting dentures, missing teeth, poor eyesight, or fatigue.

Surprisingly, monitors show little ability to compensate for their verbal production deficits by cueing the listener into their communicative intentions. Mainly they correct and revise their utterances until they hit the target or change the subject. Some may attempt to substitute another word for the target word they cannot produce, but they become so involved in correcting and revising to produce the substitution that the intent of their message is not communicated. The most likely compensatory behavior of such patients is to attempt to write or spell orally a desired word. If pushed to the limit some patients may give up and simply show the clinician with a gesture what they are trying to say.

Treatment   Conversational interaction with the monitor is easier than with the rambler. The tendency to correct and revise utterances provides opportunities for the clinician to intervene to smooth out and/or rechannel the interaction. The primary task of treatment is to keep the conversation flowing and to prevent the monitor from putting too much nonproductive effort into the correction process. One way of maintaining conversational flow is to make a verification statement when the client has conveyed his or her message with a related or an approximated word even though the actual production is an error. For example, the patient may say "I only drink blat toffee in the morning." The clinician can decrease the likelihood of the conversation being interrupted by using a verification statement such as "Black coffee— I take it that way myself."

When listening to the monitor, the clinician will need to recognize when the patient's self-correction efforts are likely to be successful and when they will lead to prolonged struggle, consequently hindering communication. When success is likely to result, it is advisable to allow the process to continue, and then to verify and/or compliment the patient. In the latter case, the clinician can fill in the missing word, and perhaps terminate the correction sequence. In making these decisions it may be helpful to keep a record of past utterances and situations in which the patient's self-correction efforts were successful and unsuccessful.

Finally, the monitor may become a better communicator when encouraged to use gestures and verbal descriptions as self-cues. Pantomiming the catching of a ball may prompt the desired word "baseball" or convey the concept to the listener. Describing the concept with statements such as "nine men" or "Babe Ruth" may accomplish the same thing. The clinician can alert the patient when it might be helpful to use these techniques with requests to "Tell me more about it" or Can you show me?" Finally, the clinician can use these techniques in his or her own speech and highlight their usefulness to the patient.

Style 3: The Unknowing Compensator

The communication style of this fluent aphasic client is one of the more interesting I have observed. The disposition of some of these cases can be tragic inasmuch as the patients devalue their ability to communicate because of the limited content of their language. Some who have experienced failure in traditional treatment paradigms may withdraw from communication entirely. The unknowing compensator scores high in concern for comprehension and does particularly well in situations having a high degree of contextual redundancy, and less well on single words and situations in which the benefits of context are denied. Yet they stand out as good listeners because of their attentiveness, and their reasonable requests for repetition and explanation.

The conversational speech of these patients is often described as "empty." These clients may refer to their hometown as "the place where I live" and to breakfast as "what I have every morning." Utterances are produced fluently with few production errors. There is little overt indication of intrapersonal monitoring, but this behavior is deceiving, because unknowing compensators actually pay very close attention to what they say and skillfully avoid the use of specific words that may require self-correction. These patients can be distinguished from anomic patients and high level conduction aphasics by their near-total lack of responsiveness to prompts and cues.

The interpersonal monitoring abilities of the unknowing compensator are excellent. These patients seem considerate and sensitive and arouse sympathy in every clinician. They show a keen awareness of the emotional aspects of the situation. They are concerned about the words missing from their speech. Some may carry on a scrap of paper a list of key words they use frequently. If they should happen to produce one of these words, they are usually elated with the result, but readily admit that they will not be able to say it again.

The most noticeable attribute of the unknowing compensators pertains to their comments about their linguistic deficits. Some patients may sound depressed. Others are self-condemning when they are unable to say frequently used words, such as a child's name or their first name.

The compensatory efforts of these patients are productive, however. They may show a listener what they want through gestures or by drawing a picture. They are particularly good at getting the listener to supply missing words or to ask questions. One of the more vivid examples I remember was an unknowing compensator trying to tell me that he had had to use insecticide to rid his home of a certain kind of pest. The following exchange took place:

Clinician: *"How has it been going with you?"*
Patient: *"Oh, not so good. I had some, you know, ughs in my place."*
Clinician: *"Ughs?"*
Patient: *"Oh, I can't say it. I can show you. It's this* (points to ear) *and then it's this* (points to head, which is bald); *I don't have one but I could use one."*
Clinician: *"Something about the ear?"*
Patient: *"Yeah, that's it, and then it's this* (points to bald head again); *I told you I need one but I haven't got one."*
Clinician: *"Your head, hair, of course, earwigs?"*
Patient: *"That's the one. I got them. Like this."* (demonstrates spraying)

Such exchanges are not unusual between unknowing compensators and listeners who are willing to allow the patient to communicate without demanding specific words. Unfortunately, patients do not always realize how well they communicate and spend their time feeling bad about their problems with specific word production.

Treatment   The management techniques that are helpful to the unknowing compensator should be obvious. They include strong psychological support, and reassurance that the patient's thoughts can be conveyed, even though specific words may be missing. As the clinician and others become more proficient in understanding such patients, they may try to "sneak in" some work on specific words, especially the words the patients badly want to say. This approach virtually always seems to result in failure, and the effort put forth does not justify the result. Treatment of the unknowing compensator should always be communication centered.

The PACE (Promoting Aphasics' Communicative Effectiveness) treatment approach devised by Davis and Wilcox (1981) provides the client with the opportunity to use all communication channels and may be helpful with the unknowing compensator. With PACE, the clinician provides immediate feedback to the patients, informing them that they are getting their message across in other ways. It is also helpful to utilize settings outside the treatment room—in stores, in barber shops, on the telephone, at the job—to demonstrate to patients how well they can do when communication, rather than specific word production, is the goal. Effort is also directed to increase the number of times a patient initiates communicative interactions.

Generally, unknowing compensators profit from treatment, not in terms of increased content word production, but in the increased awareness that they are not as helpless as they had believed. One of the positive outgrowths of the treatment of such patients is increased participation in a number of the social activities that were previously avoided.

ACCOUNTABILITY

Fluent aphasic clients have problems producing specific words; some may have difficulties understanding standard instructions or difficulty in situations with minimal contextual redundancy. They respond best to treatment approaches in which communication is "the name of the game" but may react adversely to formal testing situations in which their language deficits become readily visible. It is not a simple task to administer formal tests such as the Porch Index of Communicative Ability (PICA) (Porch, 1967) or the Boston Diagnostic Aphasia Exam (Goodglass and Kaplan, 1972) to some fluent aphasic clients. Although these instruments provide information about the client's performance on selected tasks, the clinician is often left with the feeling that the patient is really a better communicator than performance on the test indicates.

Fortunately, tools for assessing improvement are available that minimize the patient's need to perform such specific tasks as repetition, sentence completion, naming, or writing to dictation. In a test recently developed by Holland (1980a), called the Communication Abilities in Daily Living (CADL), the examiner gives the client credit for conveying information regardless of the modality employed. Also in the CADL the tester can give partial credit for responses that with a minor adjustment might be interpreted as correct. The examiner and the patient assume different roles; the former is encouraged to role play and to provide the patient with the needed contextual redundancy to show his or her skills as a communicator.

It is helpful to record portions of the treatment sessions of fluent clients. These sessions are subsequently analyzed, to determine which situations enabled the client to show increased facility with language. Often the family can provide additional information in this regard.

INVOLVEMENT OF SIGNIFICANT OTHERS

The need to involve other persons in the management of the fluent client cannot be overemphasized. The successful communications that take place between clinician and client have limited value unless extended into the environment to include spouse, co-workers, and friends. The clinician assumes responsibility for determining what facilitates and what inhibits communication, but family and friends are responsible for making communication a reality. They need to know that they must make allowances when speaking and listening to the patient so that the individual's dignity is not compromised. This point can best be made with a demonstration. The clinician should invite the family member(s) into the treatment session and explain how to talk to the patient, what to accept and what to reject, and what the patient must do to develop successfully communication skills.

CONCLUSIONS

Fluent aphasic clients do not always respond well to traditional stimulus-response paradigms. I have suggested that some fluent aphasics profit from treatment that centers on facilitating information exchange within natural communicative interactions. I have also suggested that an analysis of the communication style used by the patient may be useful in this regard. I hope that this approach will not be misinterpreted to indicate that all the clinician needs to do in treatment is to "sit down with fluent clients and have a conversation with them." Management of the fluent aphasias is complex and involves discriminative listening, interpreting, and necessary adjustment in message delivery to avoid overloading the patient's auditory system. With such patients, the clinician makes constant decisions of when to speak, listen, fill in, pause, and switch topics, to keep the interaction moving. This activity is very hard work, and its results are not always precisely measured with standardized techniques. It demands flexibility from both the clinician and the patient to succeed.

REFERENCES

Basso, A., Capitani, E., and Vignolo, L. A. 1979. Influence of rehabilitation on language skills in aphasic patients: A controlled study. Arch. Neurol. 36:190–196.

Benson, D. F. 1967. Fluency in aphasia: Correlation with radioactive scan localization. Cortex 3:373–394.

Benson, D. F. 1979. Aphasia rehabilitation: Editorial. Arch. Neurol. 36:187–189.

Beyn, E. S., and Shokhor-Trotskaya, M. K. 1966. The preventive method of speech rehabilitation in aphasia. Cortex 2:96–108.

Broida, H. 1977. Language therapy effects in long term aphasia. Arch. Phys. Med. Rehab. 58:248–253.

Dabul, B., and Bollier, B. 1976. Therapeutic approaches to apraxia. J. Speech Hear. Disord. 41:268–276.

Davis, G. A., and Wilcox, M. J. 1981. Incorporating parameters of natural conversation in aphasia treatment. In: R. Chapey (ed.), Language Intervention Strategies in Adult Aphasia. Williams & Wilkins, Baltimore.

Deal, J., and Florance, C. 1978. Modification of the eight-step continuum for treatment of apraxia of speech in adults. J. Speech Hear. Disord. 43:89–95.

Editorial. 1977. Prognosis in aphasia. Lancet 2:24.

Goodglass, H. 1981. The syndromes of aphasia: Similarities and differences in neurolinguistic features. Topics Lang. Disord. 4:1–15.

Goodglass, H., and Kaplan, E. 1972. The Assessment of Aphasia and Related Disorders. Lea & Febiger, Philadelphia.

Hagen, C. 1973. Communication abilities in hemiplegia: Effect of speech therapy. Arch. Phys. Med. Rehab. 54:454–463.

Helm, N., and Barresi B. 1980. Voluntary control of involuntary utterances: A treatment approach for severe aphasia. In: R. L. Brookshire (ed.), Clinical Aphasiology: Conference Proceedings. BRK Publishers, Minneapolis.

Helm-Estabrooks, N., Fitzpatrick, P. M., and Barresi, B. 1981. Response of an agrammatic patient to a syntax stimulation program for aphasia. J. Speech Hear. Disord. 46:422–427.

Holland, A. 1977. Some practical considerations in aphasia rehabilitation. In: M. Sullivan and M. S. Kommers (eds.), Rationale for Adult Aphasia Therapy. University of Nebraska Press, Lincoln.

Holland, A. 1980a. CADL: Communication Abilities in Daily Living. University Park Press, Baltimore.

Holland, A. 1980b. The usefulness of treatment for aphasia: A serendipitous study. In: R. L. Brookshire (ed.), Clinical Aphasiology: Conference Proceedings. BRK Publishers, Minneapolis.

Kertesz, A. 1979. Aphasia and Associated Disorders. Grune & Stratton, New York.

Kertesz, A., and McCabe, P. 1977. Recovery patterns and prognosis in aphasia. Brain 100:1–18.

Kushner, D., and Winitz, H. 1977. Extended comprehension practice applied to an aphasic patient. J. Speech Hear. Disord. 42:296–306.

Lecours, A. R., Osborn, E., Travis, L., et al. 1981. Jargons. In: J. Brown (ed.), Jargonaphasia. Academic Press, New York.

Love, R. J., and Webb, W. G. 1977. The efficacy of cueing techniques in Broca's aphasia. J. Speech Hear. Disord. 42:170–178.

Marshall, R. C. 1976. Word retrieval behavior of aphasic adults. J. Speech Hear. Disord. 41:444–451.

Marshall, R. C., and Tompkins, C. A. 1982. Verbal self-corrections of fluent and nonfluent aphasic subjects. Brain Lang. 15:292–306.

Marshall, R. C., Tompkins, C. A., and Phillips, D. S. 1982. Improvement in treated aphasia: Examination of selected prognostic factors. Folia Phoniatrica. 34:305–315.

Martin, A. D. 1981. Therapy with jargonaphasics. In: J. Brown (ed.), Jargonaphasia. Academic Press, New York.

Naeser, M. A. 1975. A structured approach teaching aphasics basic sentence types. Br. J. Commun. Disord. 10:70–76.

Porch, B. E. 1967. Porch Index of Communicative Ability. Consulting Psychologists, Palo Alto, Calif.

Rosenbek, J. C., Collins, M. J., and Wertz, R. T. 1976. Intersystemic reorganization for apraxia of speech. In: R. L. Brookshire (ed.), Clinical Aphasiology: Conference Proceedings. BRK Publishers, Minneapolis.

Rosenbek, J., Lemme, M., Ahern, M., Harris, E., and Wertz, R. 1973. A treatment for apraxia of speech in adults. J. Speech Hear. Disord. 38:462–472.

Sarno, M. T., and Levita, E. 1979. Recovery in treated aphasia in the first year post-stroke. Stroke 10:663–670.

Simmons, N. N., and Zorthian, A. 1979. Use of symbolic gestures in a case of fluent aphasia. In: R. L. Brookshire (ed.), Clinical Aphasiology: Conference Proceedings. BRK Publishers, Minneapolis.

Sparks, R., Helm, N., and Albert, M. 1974. Aphasia rehabilitation resulting from Melodic Intonation Therapy. Cortex 10:303–316.

Wepman, J. M. 1958. The relationship between self-correction and recovery from aphasia. J. Speech Hear. Disord. 23:302–305.

Wepman, J. M. 1972. Aphasia therapy: A new look. J. Speech Hear. Disord. 37:203–214.

Wertz, R. T., Kitselman, K. P., and Deal, L. A. 1981. Classifying the aphasias: Methods, prognostic implications, and efficacy of treatment. Paper presented at the Annual Convention of the American Speech-Language-Hearing Association, Los Angeles.

Wertz, R. T., Collins, M. J., Weiss, D., et al. 1982. Veterans Administration Cooperative Study of Aphasia: A comparison of individual and group treatment. J. Speech Hear. Res. 24:580–594.

Whitney, J. 1975. Developing aphasics' use of compensatory strategies. Paper presented at the convention of the American Speech and Hearing Association, Washington D.C.

CHAPTER 11

Minor Hemisphere Mediation in Aphasia Treatment

Jennifer Horner and *Karen Hardin Fedor*

Participation of the unimpaired minor hemisphere in the treatment of Broca's and Wernicke's aphasias is described by Horner and Fedor. Modalities from this hemisphere are paired with those from the dominant hemisphere, a procedure the authors believe will facilitate the restoration of language.

1. "Deblocking" is a special kind of rehabilitative approach in the treatment of aphasic patients. Define this term. Indicate whether this term refers to intrasystemic reorganization or intersystemic reorganization. What are the three kinds of deblocker that Horner and Fedor describe?

2. Distinguish between the functions of the dominant hemisphere and those of the minor hemisphere. Carefully note the difference between linguistic and ideographic functions. Why do the authors suggest that novel pictographs can enhance minor hemisphere activity?

3. What is meant by minor hemisphere participation in the treatment of aphasia? In your answer, distinguish between Broca's aphasia and Broca's aprosodia, and between Wernicke's aphasia and Wernicke's aprosodia, and describe the speech and language impairments for each of these four disorders.

4. What are the clinical deblocking procedures for the facilitation of receptive and expressive language? Are these procedures difficult to implement?

Funded, in part, by the Axe-Houghton Foundation, New York.

5. *Do you regard the clinical procedure used in minor hemisphere mediation for the treatment of aphasia to be basically different from standard clinical practices? Answer this question by considering the utilization of nonlinguistic processes in language training, the order in which linguistic units and vocal responses are trained, and the relation between receptive and expressive modalities with special regard to Broca's and Wernicke's aphasias.*

A CURRENT APPROACH TO LANGUAGE REMEDIATION for aphasia in adults involves systemic reorganization. Reorganization is possible because the capacity for linguistic operations in the aphasic individual is almost always partially spared. The goal of treatment is to access these competencies so that intelligible, informative, and pragmatically flexible communicative behaviors can be *stimulated* and/or *retrained*.

A general reorganization technique is "deblocking," that is, the deliberate pairing of an impaired function (or modality) with a relatively preserved function to facilitate performance in the impaired function. Deblocking can be intrasystemic or intersystemic. The term "function" refers to any executive behavior (Luria, 1963). In the context of aphasia treatment, we use "function" to refer to all behaviors that participate in the communicative act. "Functions" that contribute to meaningful communication are constrained by the emotional, intellectual, pragmatic, and linguistic abilities of each individual and may be automatic or volitional, paralinguistic or linguistic. When paired behaviors belong to the same functional system, treatment is called "intrasystemic reorganization." For example, a patient may be unable to imitate, but able to read aloud. The clinical technique of deblocking might involve stimulating speech through oral reading followed immediately by imitation. Then, the printed stimulus (e.g., single printed words) can be faded from the task. By pairing printed words and speech there can be "deblocking" of a "block" between auditory and oral-verbal language systems, thereby facilitating imitation of spoken language (Ulatowska and Richardson, 1974).

When paired modalities belong to different functional systems, treatment is called "intersystemic reorganization." Intersystemic reorganization involves introducing into the act of speaking a new behavior or set of behaviors in unprecedented form or with unprecedented regularity (Rosenbek, 1978, p. 195). For example, patients who are unable to imitate speech may be able to perform meaningful gestures. In some patients oral expression is facilitated when a gesture is performed immediately before a speech attempt or when both are performed simultaneously. The clinical technique of deblocking in this instance involves teaching the patient to perform a limb or manual gesture (e.g., movements showing drinking, sleeping, greetings), and then systematically to pair the imitative speech attempt with the gestural production. The gesture can be faded when the oral production is stable. In this way, a "block" between the auditory and oral-verbal language systems (i.e., impaired imitation) may be "deblocked" by pairing meaningful gestures and speech (Skelly, et al., 1974).

As discussed so far, the pairing of different language functions or modalities provides for intrasystemic reorganization, and the pairing of language and nonlanguage functions or modalities provides for intersystemic reorganization. These pairing procedures are called deblocking techniques. Another clinically relevant distinction is that between intrahemispheric and interhemispheric reorganization. Most traditional treatment approaches to aphasia use auditory stimulation. The use of intensive repetitive auditory stimulation was recognized in the early aphasia treatment literature as the cornerstone of multimodality language retraining in aphasic persons (Schuell, Jenkins, and Jiménez-Pabón, 1964). We consider this approach to be essentially intrahemispheric because it uses language to treat language. More specifically, traditional approaches focus on phonologic-semantic-syntactic behaviors, with an assumption that comprehension ("reauditorization") precedes expression during language recovery.

Within the past decade, several innovative approaches for the treatment of aphasia have been developed. They include the use of melody (Sparks, Helm, and Albert, 1974), novel pictographic stimuli (Gardner et al., 1976), visual imagery (West, 1978), and action (Helm and Benson, 1978). These approaches are fundamentally different from the traditional approaches to aphasia treatment because they are nonlinguistic. Specifically, these new approaches use holistic and nonphonetic stimuli to facilitate language. We consider these approaches to be interhemispheric deblocking techniques because behaviors recognized to be functions of the minor hemisphere are being used to facilitate linguistic communication.

This chapter presents a systematic model of interhemispheric deblocking of aphasic language. To this end, the neuropsychological attributes of the dominant hemisphere, usually the left hemisphere, and the minor hemisphere, usually the right hemisphere, are reviewed. Additionally, several techniques for remediation are described. These techniques involve the use of affective-prosodic, visual-spatial-holistic, and rudimentary linguistic stimuli.

PARTICIPATION OF DOMINANT AND MINOR HEMISPHERES IN COMMUNICATION

Visual-spatial and other nonverbal functions are ascribed to the minor hemisphere, whereas language functions are ascribed to the dominant hemisphere in most adults (Searleman, 1977; Moscovitch, 1976, 1981). In this regard, the hemispheres of the brain are "asymmetrical" in terms of their primary functions.

Table 1 reviews the distinctive and complementary communicative functions of the dominant and minor hemispheres. The two cerebral hemispheres differ not only in their respective capacities for language, but also in their strategies or modes of operation in processing language. The dominant hemisphere is predisposed to use phonetic, sequential, and analytic-perceptual cognitive strategies; the minor hemisphere is geared for visual-spatial and holistic strategies. The aptitudes of the dominant hemisphere, which are predominantly *linguistic* (symbolic), include the ability to recognize and formulate messages through the rule based selection and sequencing of sounds and words. The aptitudes of the minor hemisphere are predominantly *ideographic*. Ideographic processing refers to the ability to derive meaning (an idea or a concept) directly or holistically from a stimulus, as distinguished

Table 1.   Participation of dominant (left) and minor (right) hemispheres in the communication processes

Dominant hemisphere	Minor hemisphere
Processes	
Phonetic-sequential-analytic	Visual-spatial-holistic
Aptitudes	
Linguistic	Ideographic
(Symbolic)	(Affective, melodic, enactive)
Phonologic rules	Facial expression
Syntactic rules	Emotional gestures
Lexical-semantic rules	Tone of voice
Shared aptitudes	
Verbal memory	
Comprehension of concrete, imageable, operative, and emotional words	
Comprehension of basic syntax	
Functions	
Auditory comprehension of word order	Auditory comprehension of affective-prosodic changes (tone of voice)
Spontaneous expression of ideas via words and sentences	Spontaneous expression of ideas via prosody and emotional gesturing
Repetition of words and sentences	Repetition of prosody and emotional gestures
Visual graphemic expression of ideas (writing)	Visual-pictographic expression of ideas (copying-drawing)
Visual comprehension of printed words (analytic-phonic strategy)	Visual comprehension of printed words (holistic strategy)
	Visual comprehension of emotional gestures of face and arms

from feature-by-feature analysis (e.g., sound-by-sound or letter-by-letter strategies). An ideograph may be a facial expression (e.g., a frown), an intonation pattern (e.g., a question), or an action (e.g., bowing the head, clenching a fist). We refer to these as affective, melodic, and enactive ideographs, respectively. Aptitudes thought to be shared by both hemispheres include verbal memory and comprehension of words and basic sentences (Zaidel, 1978). In particular, words that are highly familiar (concrete words), words that evoke visual images (imageable words), words that are associated with actions or manipulations (operative words), and words that are used to convey emotions (emotional words) have been shown to be recognizable by both hemispheres.

Some researchers have suggested that the minor hemisphere is capable of assuming language function in the event of dominant hemisphere lesions (Kinsbourne, 1971; Cummings et al., 1979). Others have added that specific modes of stimulation may enhance minor hemisphere participation. Clinicians have been encouraged to "tap the minor hemisphere" in aphasia treatment through the use of verbs of motion and manipulation (Gardner, 1973), and visual imaging (West, 1978). Verbs that are familiar and involve manipulation of objects or bodily movements are recommended—for example, get, do, make, climb, sit, move (West, 1978).

Our understanding of the concept of "imaging" is important to our selection of stimulus materials in aphasia treatment if we are to "tap the minor hemisphere." Myers (1980, p. 69) defines an image as ". . . a nonverbal confluence of emotion, intellect and sensation." To evoke "images"—and thereby engage the minor hemisphere—it is recommended that stimulus pictures used in aphasia treatment depict not only simple actions, but also *interactive relationships* among people and objects. Stimulus pictures should include meaningful contexts and also should *require an interpretation* by the patient (Myers, 1980). Because the minor hemisphere is specialized for the synthesis and interpretation of multiple relationships, Myers recommends the use of elaborated pictorial stimuli. Simple action pictures alone are less likely to stimulate "imaging" than pictures showing interactions among people and objects (e.g., a man intently watching a football game on television or a man giving directions to another man). Imaging is further heightened when such interactions are depicted in meaningful settings (e.g., a man intently watching a football game on television with newspapers strewn about the room, or a man giving another man directions on a busy street corner during a rainstorm).

"Novelty" may also enhance minor hemisphere participation in language (Faber and Aten, 1979; Gardner et al., 1976; Horner and LaPointe, 1979). Novel pictographs, such as Blissymbolics, can enhance minor hemisphere activity because they are visual, static, and nonphonetic (Horner and LaPointe, 1979). The visual aspect bypasses the auditory processing deficit inherent in aphasia; the static feature minimizes the memory load inherent in temporally ordered auditory stimuli, and the feature of novelty minimizes the patient's tendency to respond in a "biased" and erroneous manner to previously known material (Goldberg and Costa, 1981; Winitz, 1969). It has also been suggested that so-called ideographic abilities, such as recognition of familiar printed words and gestures, are retained in some aphasic individuals (Heilman and Rothi, 1980; Zaidel and Peters, 1981).

Thus, minor hemisphere participation may be enhanced by careful selection of treatment stimuli. Several dimensions recognized to be of value in this regard are picturability, familiarity, manipulability, interactive imagery, interpretive complexity, and novelty. In general, the use of nonverbal stimuli that may enhance holistic-ideographic mental processing and imaging is recommended when developing an interhemispheric deblocking treatment program.

Minor Hemisphere Participation in Language Acquisition

Language maturation—and the concomitant emergence of functional hemispheric asymmetries—are life-long processes (Brown and Hecaen, 1976). Studies of neuropsychological maturation suggest that the hemispheres are equally involved in prelingual perceptual-cognitive development necessary to language emergence. As early as the first or second year of life, the left hemisphere assumes a dominant role in language acquisition and the right hemisphere becomes less significantly involved (Annett, 1973). However, recent research suggests that the minor hemisphere *retains an essential role in the elaboration and execution of symbolic thought throughout the language maturation process*. For example, extralinguistic functions subserved by the minor hemisphere may include appreciation of thematic, connotative, humorous, and pragmatic aspects of communication (Moscovitch, 1981). The minor hemisphere participates in the early language acquisition process, also playing an essential role in the life-long maturation process. This is an important consideration for our model of aphasia treatment. The phenomenon suggests that the minor hemisphere may mediate language recovery in individuals with acquired aphasia. These considerations provide a background for the interhemispheric model proposed here. As clinicians of aphasic patients, we need to consider *the selection and manipulation of stimuli that will engage minor hemisphere participation to rehabilitate the language functions of the aphasic person.*

The Aphasias and the Aprosodias

Studies of right hemisphere stroke patients indicate that the minor hemisphere governs the expression and comprehension of affect conveyed through facial expression and vocal prosody and body gestures. For example, Heilman, Scholes, and Watson (1975) found disturbed comprehension of affective speech (affective agnosia) in right hemisphere damaged patients, a finding corroborated by others, including Ross (1981).

Ross (1981) drew an analogy between dominant hemisphere aphasias and minor hemisphere "aprosodias" (Table 2). For example, an anterior minor hemisphere lesion resulted in *motor* (Broca's) *aprosodia*, which is characterized by: 1) spontaneously flat tone of voice and facial expression, 2) inability to repeat phrases with tones of voice representing angry, sad, happy, and so on, and 3) retained ability to recognize the speaker's affective intent by the tone of his voice. *Motor* (Broca's) *aphasia*, by comparison, is characterized by: 1) short, hesitant, and amelodic utterances, 2) effortful initiation, hesitancy, and sound substitutions, and 3) retained ability to understand spoken language (Ross, 1981, p. 564). Thus, from the study of acquired neuropsychological deficits in both right and left hemisphere damaged patients, Ross (1981) proposes the following model: 1) the left (dominant) hemisphere is the center for linguistic-propositional communication, 2) the right (minor) hemisphere is the center for prosodic-affective communication, and 3) the anterior cortex of both hemispheres subserves expressive functions while the posterior cortex of both hemispheres subserves receptive functions.

FACILITATION AND REORGANIZATION OF APHASIA THROUGH MINOR HEMISPHERE MEDIATION

Minor hemispheric mediation as a language remediation approach encompasses two major goals: facilitation and reorganization of the *receptive* language functions of the dominant hemisphere, and facilitation and reorganization of the *expressive* language functions of the dominant hemisphere. Underlying this approach are the assumptions that under appropriate stimulus conditions, the minor hemisphere can be tapped to mediate language recovery, and that the potential for linguistic (phonologic, syntactic, and semantic) recovery can be enhanced through systematic pairing of expressive and receptive communicative behaviors with ideographic stimuli that engage minor hemisphere perceptual-cognitive processes (Horner, 1983).

Table 2. Neuropsychologic deficits of the dominant and minor hemispheres

Functions	Dominant hemisphere linguistic deficits		Minor hemisphere prosodic-affective deficits[a]	
	Broca's (anterior) aphasia	Wernicke's (posterior) aphasia	Broca's (anterior) aprosodia	Wernicke's (posterior) aprosodia
Spontaneous speech	Nonfluent agrammatic speech	Fluent, paraphasic speech	Aprosodic-agestural speech	Prosodic-gestural speech
Comprehension	Relatively preserved comprehension	Impaired comprehension	Good comprehension of prosody and emotional gestures	Poor comprehension of prosody and emotional gestures
Repetition	Impaired repetition	Impaired repetition	Poor prosodic repetition	Poor prosodic repetition

[a] Ross (1981).

Facilitation and Reorganization of Receptive Language

Deblocking Receptive Aphasia Using Minor Hemisphere Mediation The physiologic aspects of dominant and minor hemisphere interaction involve two principal routes (Berlin, 1976): 1) Transcallosal pathways are interhemispheric and connect homologous areas of both hemispheres; that is, Broca's area in the dominant hemisphere is connected via transcallosal pathways with the homologue to Broca's area in the minor hemisphere, and dominant Wernicke's area is connected with its homologue in the minor hemisphere. 2) Posterior-to-anterior (and anterior-to-posterior) pathways connect areas within the same hemisphere via the large tract of fibers called the arcuate fasciculus. These connections are intrahemispheric and occur in both hemispheres (Figure 1). In individuals with a significant receptive aphasic disorder (usually, Wernicke's aphasia) due to a lesion in the auditory association area of the dominant hemisphere, an interhemispheric mediation or "deblocking" of receptive dysfunction is possible using these pathways as shown in Figure 2. In this approach, deblocking of auditory comprehension can begin with stimulation of minor hemisphere expressive *or* receptive skills. When expression is stimulated, intact anterior-to-posterior pathways transfer information from minor Broca's area to minor Wernicke's area, where transcallosal fibers then relay input to the dominant Wernicke's area. When minor hemisphere receptive skills are stimulated, transcallosal fibers transfer the information directly to the dominant Wernicke's area.

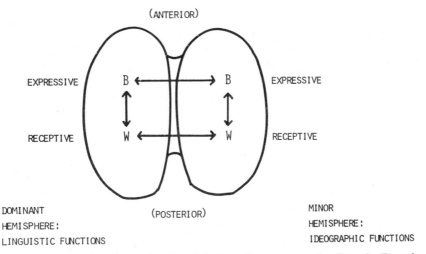

Figure 1. Normal intra- and interhemispheric pathways connecting Broca's (B) and Wernicke's (W) areas of the dominant (left) and minor (right) hemispheres.

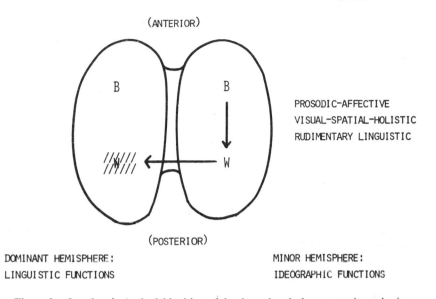

Figure 2.   Interhemispheric deblocking of dominant hemisphere receptive aphasia.

The purpose of minor hemisphere mediation treatment of receptive dysfunction is to "deblock" (access, stimulate, and/or retrain) auditory comprehension. This deblocking is accomplished by pairing intact minor hemisphere capacities with impaired dominant hemisphere functions. The goal is to improve attention to, and comprehension of, spoken messages.

At least three types of "deblocker" of minor hemisphere origin are available for linguistic stimulation of the dominant hemisphere. These are visual-spatial-holistic, affective-prosodic, and rudimentary linguistic. In Table 3, which gives deblocking treatments for receptive aphasia, the "mode of prestimulation" designates whether the deblocking information is *directly* tapped via minor Wernicke's area (direct receptive deblocking) or *indirectly* tapped via minor Broca's area (indirect expressive-to-receptive deblocking).

As with other treatment programs, the clinician should control the linguistic complexity of the input by restricting length, using familiar vocabulary, and simplifying syntactic structure. Although we individualize instruction, it is our opinion that direct treatment of receptive language can be terminated as soon as the patient is able to attend to the clinician and to follow task instructions that are used in subsequent phases of treatment that focus on the reorganization of expressive language. In this way, the majority of the treatment effort can be directed to expressive language. Of course, the receptive language performance

Table 3. Deblocking of receptive aphasic disorders using minor hemisphere mediation

Linguistic goal	Type of deblocker	Mode of prestimulation	Technique
To facilitate attention to, discrimination of, and comprehension of spoken messages (words, sentences, and discourse)	Visual-spatial-holistic	Receptive	Clinican presents a gesture, then a spoken word as patient watches and listens
			Clinician presents a novel symbol, then a spoken word as patient watches and listens
		Expressive	Clinician presents a gesture, then a spoken word; patient imitates the gesture and listens
			Clinician presents a picture or a word to be copied then a spoken word; patient draws and listens
	Affective-prosodic	Receptive	Clinician uses emotionally toned prosodic patterns concurrently with speech as patient listens
			Clinician uses diverse facial expressions concurrently with speech as patient watches and listens
		Expressive	Clinician presents an emotional gesture and facial expression; patient imitates the emotional gesture and facial expression and listens to the spoken message
	Rudimentary linguistic	Receptive	Clinician presents a printed word amenable to ideographic processing concurrently with speech; patient reads silently or aloud, or listens as clinician reads aloud
		Expressive	Clinician dictates a whole word to be written; patient writes the word and listens to the spoken message

of each patient influences the clinician's choice of deblocker and mode of prestimulation throughout the treatment program.

Facilitation and Reorganization of Expressive Language

With regard to the physiology of interhemispheric and intrahemispheric transfer of information, Berlin (1976) has offered some guidelines for the treatment of language expression. If the posterior-anterior arcuate fasciculus is disrupted (as is likely in patients with impaired repetition; see Table 2), he suggested that the accessing and monitoring of spontaneous speech be done via the *minor Broca's area*. This approach would apply to both the nonfluent, agrammatic speech of Broca's aphasia and the fluent but paraphasic speech of Wernicke's aphasia, which is characterized by semantic (word selection) and phonemic (sound selection) errors. According to this approach, minor hemisphere posterior-anterior pathways and minor-to-dominant transcallosal pathways are regarded as intact (see Figures 3 and 4). In Broca's aphasia, interhemispheric deblocking engages minor hemisphere functions for receptive and expressive language, with supplemental input from the receptive and expressive areas of the dominant hemisphere. Final speech output is then executed by the dominant Broca's area via the minor Broca's area (Figure 3). In Wernicke's aphasia, supplemental

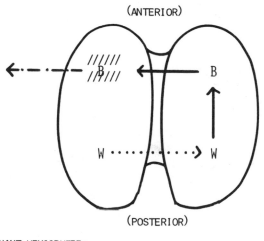

(ANTERIOR)

(POSTERIOR)

DOMINANT HEMISPHERE: MINOR HEMISPHERE:
LINGUISTIC FUNCTIONS   IDEOGRAPHIC FUNCTIONS

Figure 3.   In Broca's aphasia, interhemispheric deblocking engages minor hemisphere functions both receptive and expressive (solid arrow), with supplemental input from dominant hemisphere receptive and expressive areas (dotted arrow). Final speech output is executed by the dominant Broca's area via the minor Broca's area (dash–dot arrow).

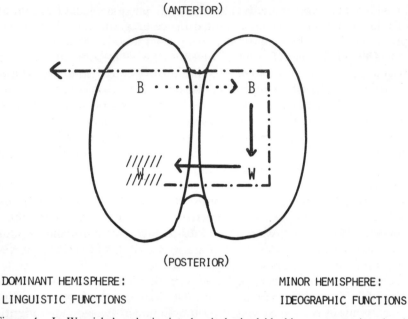

Figure 4. In Wernicke's aphasia, interhemispheric deblocking engages minor hemisphere functions, both receptive and expressive (solid arrow). Supplemental input from dominant hemisphere Broca's area (dotted arrows) joins with minor hemisphere functions. Final speech output is routed through the minor hemisphere via transcallosal pathways to the dominant Broca's area (dash–dot arrow).

input from the dominant Broca's area joins with the minor hemisphere functions to deblock dominant Wernicke's area deficits. Output from Wernicke's area is then routed through the minor hemisphere via transcallosal and intrahemispheric pathways to the dominant Broca's area (Figure 4).

As in the receptive deblocking model, three types of deblocker are available for expressive deficits: affective-prosodic, visual-spatial-holistic, and rudimentary linguistic. For both Broca's and Wernicke's aphasias, the focus of treatment is verbal expression. The goal is to stimulate speech that is affective, informative, and pragmatically flexible. The treatment techniques described in Tables 4 and 5 are best suited to the patient who possesses sufficient residual language in the dominant hemisphere to make pairing strategies feasible. For this reason, individuals with aphasia of moderate severity are best suited for training by minor hemisphere mediation.

Deblocking Broca's Aphasia Using Minor Hemisphere Mediation Treatment for the nonfluent, agrammatic speech of Broca's aphasia focuses on three levels of remediation, described in the order in which they are treated: 1) prosody, 2) phonology, and 3) syntax (Table 4). Within each level, linguistic goals are arranged in an approximate hierarchy of difficulty (from least to most difficult).

The syllable is the minimal unit for prosodic treatment. The first goal at this level involves establishing control of volitional phonation. It can be accomplished by pairing prosodic-affective deblockers, (emotional facial expressions), and visual-spatial-holistic deblockers, (whole body movements), with vocalization. After control of duration and tone has been achieved at the syllable level, basic intonation patterns (negation, affirmation, and interrogation) and prosodic variability at the phrase level are established using deblockers of similar types.

The word is the minimal unit of treatment at the level of phonologic treatment. The first goal of establishing single-word holophrastic utterances is addressed by using visual-spatial-holistic and rudimentary linguistic deblockers. Utterance length is then increased using visual-spatial holistic cues, such as pairing speech with symbolic gestures or novel pictorial symbols.

The phrase is the minimal unit at the level of syntactic treatment. The clinician should organize stimuli into homogeneous sets according to sentence type, form class, and length. To minimize the patient's tendency to rely on nominal forms, the clinician should treat nouns, verbs, and adjectives equally. The initial goal involves eliciting phonologic expression at the phrase level with rudimentary linguistic deblockers, such as highly familiar phrases that were acquired largely by rote memory. The next goal at this level is to establish basic sentence types in the present tense, active voice, by using visual-spatial-holistic deblockers that pair speech with sequences of symbolic gestures (e.g., "I drink water."). At subsequent stages, adjectives and negatives are introduced and sentence length is increased through concatenation, or the stringing of phrases (e.g., "The boy runs *and* the boy sings."). These goals are accomplished by using a variety of rudimentary linguistic and visual-spatial-holistic deblockers, such as ideographic reading, novel symbols, gestures, grammatical tree diagrams, and diacritical marks.

Deblocking   Wernicke's   Aphasia   Using   Minor   Hemisphere Mediation   Treatment of the fluent paraphasic speech of Wernicke's aphasia focuses on four levels of remediation: 1) prosody, 2) phonology, 3) semantics, and 4) syntax (Table 5). Within each level, linguistic goals are arranged in an approximate hierarchy of difficulty. Because of the auditory comprehension and associated self-monitoring deficits evident with Wernicke's aphasia, a treatment format that strengthens feedback skills is desirable. We recommend the use of a treatment format called "Promoting Aphasics' Communicative Effectiveness"

Table 4. Deblocking of Broca's aphasia using minor hemisphere mediation

Linguistic goal	Type of deblocker	Technique
	Treatment of prosody	
To establish control of continuous volitional phonation with control of duration and tone at the syllable level	Affective-prosodic	Pair emotional arm and face gestures with emotionally intoned voice (e.g., surprise—oh!; anger—mm!) Pair emotional facial expressions and intonations with continuous voicing, simultaneously with clinician
	Visual-spatial-holistic	Pair whole body movements with simultaneous voicing (e.g., standing up, turning, leaning forward and backward)
To establish basic intonation patterns (e.g., negation, affirmation, interrogation) at the holophrastic level	Affective-prosodic	Pair facial expression with emotionally intoned single words (e.g., negation—no; affirmation—yes; interrogation—what?)
To establish prosodic variability in words and phrases of increasing length; to move primary stress gradually from initial to medial to final position	Visual-spatial-holistic	Pair gross body movements with prosodic changes in stress, duration, and pause (e.g., vertical arm movements corresponding to changes in stress; horizontal arm movements corresponding to changes in duration and pause) Using horizontal and vertical line drawings to represent visually pause and stress variation, respectively; clinician has patient trace line patterns with finger as clinician simultaneously voices (hums or produces prolonged vowels) in the designated prosodic pattern

Treatment of phonology

Goal		Treatment
To establish single-word holophrastic utterances	Visual-spatial-holistic	Pair speech with static gestures (e.g., up, down, go, what)
To increase utterance length	Rudimentary linguistic	Stimulate automatic speech, recitation, and expletives
	Visual-spatial-holistic	Pair speech with symbolic gestures, such as signing through Ameslan for hunger, bathroom, water, etc. Pair speech with novel pictorial symbols

Treatment of syntax

Goal		Treatment
To establish phonologic-prosodic expression at the phrase level	Rudimentary linguistic	Stimulate frequently used phrases that may be automatic (e.g., How are you? Time to go)
To establish basic sentence types in the present tense, active voice, emphasizing verbs of motion	Visual-spatial-holistic	Pair speech with sequences of symbolic gestures (e.g., I drink water; you go home)
To introduce adjectives and negation	Rudimentary linguistic	Pair speech with sequences of printed words amenable to whole word (ideographic) reading
	Visual-spatial-holistic	Pair speech with sequences of novel symbols. Pair speech with sequences of gestures
To increase sentence length through concatenation (e.g., The boy runs and the boy sings; The boy works and the boy is hot).	Visual-spatial-holistic	Use grammatical tree diagrams to help patient visualize form class differences and word order rules. Use diacritical marks to indicate interphrase boundaries and associated intonational changes

Table 5.   Deblocking of Wernicke's aphasia using minor hemisphere mediation

Linguistic goal	Type of deblocker	Techniques
	Treatment of prosody	
To increase volitional use of intonation contours used in spontaneous speech	Affective-prosodic	Pair appropriate facial expression with the intent of a message (e.g., a puzzled expression with a question)
		Pair appropriate emotional tone/melodic contour with the intent of the message (e.g., question vs. command vs. warning)
	Visual-spatial-holistic	Pair holistic body movements and pantomimic gestures with intent of message
		Use changes in body posture and body movement to signal turn taking
	Treatment of phonology	
To minimize phonemic paraphasic errors, neologisms, and jargon	Visual-spatial-holistic	Elicit emotional and descriptive speech with altered pictorial stimuli and contextualized actions that stimulate connotative and thematic interpretations
		Pair speech with pantomimic gestures; identify the locus of paraphasic errors in relation to these dimensions in connected speech
	Affective-prosodic	Pair speech with changes in tone of voice; identify the locus of paraphasic errors in relation to melodic contour in connected speech

Treatment of semantics

To decrease semantic paraphasias	Visual-spatial-holistic and rudimentary linguistic	Patient matches a printed word with an appropriate picture from a group of semantically related pictures, then reads the word aloud
		Patient is shown a picture, then silently reads a list of semantically related words, choosing and reading aloud the target word which is visually distinctive (e.g., bowl, cup, PLATE, glass)
	Affective-prosodic	In response to paraphasic errors, clinician reacts with changes in facial expression or gestures as signals to patient to repeat the speech attempt
	Visual-spatial-holistic	Patient selects the target word from a choice of pictures during connected speech; pictures show actions that can be labeled with verbs of motion or objects that are easily manipulated or recognized as whole body movements
		Patient draws a picture in attempting word retrieval
		Patient gestures a semantic feature (e.g., shape, size, function) then attempts word retrieval
		Patient responds to "altered" pictorial stimuli that are designed to facilitate word retrieval and descriptive word associations (e.g., "broken ladder," "bent hanger," "spilled coffee")
		Patient is instructed to recall an image ("mental picture") and retrieve the word concurrently
To increase word retrieval ability and decrease anomic gaps	Visual-spatial-holistic and rudimentary linguistic	Patient tries to write the beginning of the word, point to an alphabet display, or indicate the size and shape of the word to facilitate word retrieval

continued

Table 5. *(Continued)*

Linguistic goal	Type of deblocker	Techniques
		Treatment of syntax
To decrease paragrammatic errors	Visual-spatial-holistic and rudimentary linguistic	Pair spoken word sequences with corresponding pantomimed actions; the patient is encouraged to imitate the meaningful pantomime and then to imitate the speech-plus-pantomime sequence
		Using printed words amenable to whole word reading, present printed sentences controlled for length and sentence type
		Present printed cards, grouped in stacks by form class and organized in correct sequence; patient formulates sentences by selecting cards, left to right, then reads the sentence aloud
		Present printed sentences with blanks (e.g., "The _____ is _____ing the _____."). Patient is instructed to complete the sentence by writing or saying the missing words aloud. If anomia is severe and persistent, patient is encouraged to circumvent "anomic gaps" by substituting contentives with descriptive phrases or general terms such as "thing," "this one," or "that one."
		Using printed words amenable to whole word reading, color code the various syntactic forms (e.g., ART + N + AUX + Ving); patient first places the cards in correct order, then reads aloud

(PACE) (Davis and Wilcox, 1981). PACE is designed so that the clinician and the patient convey to each other new information in a natural conversational setting and participate equally in the roles of message sender and message receiver.

The dyadic format of PACE is advantageous because feedback about the communicative adequacy of spoken messages is enhanced. As message sender, the patient can evaluate the adequacy of his or her message by attending to the clinician's feedback. As message receiver, the patient has the opportunity to let the clinician know whether the message has been understood.

Because the profile of Wernicke's aphasia is distinctly different from that of Broca's aphasia (see Table 2), the specific treatment goals differ. However, the basic concept of minor hemisphere participation is shared by both treatments and the deblocker types are similar.

The minimal unit for treating prosodic contour and syntax in the Wernicke's aphasic is the sentence. The minimal unit for treating either phonologic or semantic form is the word in sentence context. Deblocking techniques, alone or in combination, can be applied in an eclectic manner. General techniques such as controlling pause and encouraging silent rehearsal can be readily integrated with the techniques suggested here. Written expression (copying and/or spontaneous writing) can be treated concurrently with oral-verbal expressive training.

The primary goal at the level of prosodic treatment is to increase the volitional use of intonation contours in spontaneous speech. Affective-prosodic deblockers, such as pairing appropriate facial expressions with the intent of a message, and such visual-spatial-holistic deblockers as pairing whole body movements and pantomimic gestures with the intent of a message, are effective.

The primary goal at the level of phonologic treatment is to minimize phonemic (sound) paraphasic errors, neologisms, and jargon. A number of visual-spatial-holistic cues, as described in Table 5, are considered to be facilitative.

Semantic treatment emphasizes decreasing semantic (word) paraphasic errors, increasing word retrieval ability, and decreasing anomic gaps. Semantic paraphasias can be decreased using visual-spatial-holistic deblockers that consist of printed words and pictures controlled for semantic similarity and paired with oral reading. Affective-prosodic cues provided by the clinician also give the patient feedback regarding semantic errors in his or her speech. To increase word retrieval and decrease anomic gaps, visual-spatial-holistic deblockers include picture selection, picture drawing retrieval attempts, gesturing semantic features of target units, and responding to "altered" stimuli (Faber and Aten, 1979). Rudimentary linguistic deblockers are combined with visual-spatial-holistic cues when the patient attempts to write the target word, point to an alphabetic display, or indicate size and shape of a target word as in a word retrieval effort.

Syntactic rehabilitation is the final level of treatment for the patient with Wernicke's aphasia. The principal goal at this level is to decrease paragrammatic errors, defined as the production of unacceptable word sequences, confusion of verb tense, errors in pronoun case and gender, and incorrect choice of prepositions. A number of visual-spatial-holistic and rudimentary linguistic cues can be used to decrease paragrammatic errors. Pairing speech with a sequence of pantomimic gestures is one technique. Other strategies involve pairing speech with printed words that are visually distinctive in one or more ways. Words that are color coded according to syntactic form, incomplete sentences with visual cues to sentence type and length, and words grouped in stacks by form class and organized in correct sequence, which the patient must then read aloud, are examples of combined visual-spatial-holistic and rudimentary linguistic deblockers.

SUMMARY

In describing recovery from aphasia through minor hemisphere mediation, it was asserted that the potential for linguistic recovery can be enhanced through systematic pairing of impaired linguistic behaviors with ideographic stimuli, subserved by the dominant and minor hemispheres, respectively. Three types of ideographic stimulus used as "deblocking" agents are affective-prosodic, visual-spatial-holistic, and rudimentary linguistic behaviors. A variety of tasks designed to stimulate and reorganize the language of Wernicke's and Broca's aphasias through minor hemisphere mediation were described.

REFERENCES

Annett, M. 1973. Laterality of childhood hemiplegia and the growth of speech and intelligence. Cortex. 9:4–33.

Berlin, C. I. 1976. On: Melodic Intonation Therapy for Aphasia by R. W. Sparks and A. L. Holland. J. Speech Hear. Disord. 41:298–300.

Brown, J. W., and Hecaen, H. 1976. Lateralization and language representation. Neurology 26:183–189.

Cummings, J. L., Benson, D. F., Walsh, M. J., and Levine, H. L. 1979. Left-to-right transfer of language dominance: A case study. Neurology 29:1547–1550.

Davis, G. A., and Wilcox, J. 1981. Incorporating parameters of natural conversation in aphasia treatment. In: R. Chapey (ed.), Language Intervention Strategies in Adult Aphasia. Williams & Wilkins, Baltimore.

Faber, M. M., and Aten, J. L. 1979. Verbal performance in aphasic patients in response to intact and altered pictorial stimuli. In: R. H. Brookshire (ed.), Clinical Aphasiology: Conference Proceedings, 1979, pp. 177–186. BRK Publishers, Minneapolis.

Gardner, H. 1973. The contribution of operativity to naming capacity in aphasic patients. Neuropsychologia 11:213–220.

Gardner, H., Zurif, E. G., Berry, T., and Baker, E. 1976. Visual communication in aphasia. Neuropsychologia 14:275–292.

Goldberg, E., and Costa, L. D. 1981. Hemisphere differences in the acquisition and use of descriptive systems. Brain Lang. 14:144–173.

Heilman, K. M., and Rothi, L. J. 1980. Acquired reading disorders: A diagrammatic model. Paper presented at the Sixth Annual Course in Behavioral Neurology and Neuropsychology, Daytona.

Heilman, K. M., Scholes, R., and Watson, R. T. 1975. Auditory affective agnosia. J. Neurol. Neurosurg. Psychiat. 38:69–72.

Helm, N. A., and Benson, D. F. 1978. Visual action therapy for global aphasia. Paper presented to the Academy of Aphasia, Chicago, October.

Horner, J. 1983. Treatment of Broca's aphasia: Facilitation and reorganization. In, W. H. Perkins (ed.), Current Therapy of Communication Disorders. Thieme-Stratton, New York.

Horner, J., and LaPointe, L. L. 1979. Evaluation of learning potential in a severe aphasic adult through analysis of five performance variables. In: R. H. Brookshire (ed.), Clinical Aphasiology: Conference Proceedings, 1979, pp. 101–114. BRK Publishers, Minneapolis.

Kinsbourne, M. 1971. The minor cerebral hemisphere. Arch. Neurol. 25:302–306.

Luria, A. R. 1963. Restoration of Function After Brain Injury, O. L. Zangwill (trans. ed.). Macmillan, New York.

Moscovitch, M. 1976. On the representation of language in the right hemisphere of right-handed people. Brain Lang. 3:47–71.

Moscovitch, M. 1981. Right-hemisphere language. In: P. O'Connell (ed.), Topics in Language Disorders 1:41–61.

Myers, P. 1980. Visual imagery in aphasia treatment: A new look. In: R. H. Brookshire (ed.), Clinical Aphasiology: Conference Proceedings, 1980, pp. 68–77. BRK Publishers, Minneapolis.

Rosenbek, J. C. 1978. Treating apraxia of speech. In: D. F. Johns (ed.), Clinical Management of Neurogenic Communicative Disorders, pp. 191–242. Little, Brown, Boston.

Ross, E. D. 1981. The aprosodias: Functional-anatomic organization of the affective components of language in the right hemisphere. Arch. Neurol. 38:561–569.

Schuell, H., Jenkins, J. J., and Jiménez-Pabón, E. 1964. Aphasia in Adults: Diagnosis, Prognosis and Treatment. Hoeber, New York.

Searleman, A. 1977. A review of right hemisphere linguistic capabilities. Psychol. Bull. 84:503–528.

Skelly, M., Schinsky, L., Smith, R. W., and Fust, R. S. 1974. American Indian Sign (Amerind) as a facilitator of verbalization for the oral verbal apraxic. J. Speech Hear. Disord. 39:445–456.

Sparks, R., Helm, N., and Albert, M. 1974. Aphasia rehabilitation resulting from melodic intonation therapy. Cortex 10:303–316.

Ulatowska, H. K., and Richardson, S. M. 1974. A longitudinal study of an adult with aphasia: Considerations for research and therapy. Brain Lang. 1:151–166.

West, J. F. 1978. Heightening the action imagery of materials used in aphasia treatment. In: R. H. Brookshire (ed.), Clinical Aphasiology: Conference Proceedings, 1978, pp. 201–211. BRK Publishers, Minneapolis.

Winitz, H. 1969. Articulatory Acquisition and Behavior. Appleton-Century-Crofts, New York.

Zaidel, E. 1978. Lexical organization in the right hemisphere. In: P. A. Buser and T. Roygeul-Buser (eds.), Cerebral Correlates of Conscious Experience (INSERM Symposium no. 6). Elsevier/North Holland Biomedical Press, Amsterdam.

Zaidel, E., and Peters, A. M. 1981. Phonological encoding and ideographic reading by the disconnected right hemisphere: Two case studies. Brain Lang. 14:205–234.

CHAPTER 12

Vocabulary Selection in Augmentative Communication
Where Do We Begin?

Andrea F. Blau

> *Augmentative communication systems enable the individual without oral language to communicate. Blau provides guidelines for the selection and teaching of the initial vocabulary for the nonvocal child and adult.*

1. *According to Blau, what are the qualifications when using a developmental model in the selection of lexical items for augmentative communication?*
2. *Discuss Blau's recommendations for the selection of a word pool. Which ones do you believe should be given primary attention?*
3. *What constraints, according to Blau, does the symbol system impose on the selection of items for an initial lexicon? Can you add to this list?*
4. *What is your interpretation of Blau's guidelines for the selection of a lexicon that should have the "broadest functional utility" and the "highest interest level"? Which proposals do you agree with and which do you disagree with?*
5. *Why is consideration of discourse principles important in the selection and organization of a nonspeaker's lexicon?*

Masculine pronouns are used throughout this chapter for the sake of grammatical uniformity and simplicity. They are not meant to be preferential or discriminatory.

THE DECISION MAKING PROCESSES (DMP) in augmentative communication intervention have been the focus of a new body of literature in the field of speech and language pathology. The large number of articles and workshops dealing with augmentative communication in the past 5 years, and the founding of a journal, indicate growing interest in non-vocal techniques and increasing demand for training models for speech and language clinicians.

Guidelines are currently available for the *evaluation*, *candidacy election*, *technique*, and *symbol set selection* procedures for optimally developing an augmentative system for a nonspeaking individual's unique functional needs (Chapman and Miller, 1980; Harris and Vanderheiden, 1980a; Meyers et al., 1980; Shane, 1981; Vanderheiden, 1980b). These guidelines have emphasized the enhancement of an individual's *existing* ability to interact within his environment by carefully reflecting on his physical, intellectual, sensory, perceptual, linguistic, emotional, environmental, and communicatively interpersonal concerns.

Although clinical experience supports the hypothesis that the introduction and use of augmentative communication enhances the communicative interaction skills of many nonspeaking clients, two important features of the DMP have not yet been adequately examined. These interrelated features, the *language content* of the nonspeaker's communication system and the *implementation strategies* most effective for appropriate training and efficient system use, remain in the preliminary stages of investigation.

Our lack of sophistication regarding these features is no reflection of their lack of importance in our intervention programming. In many respects, our proficiency in making appropriate decisions has evolved in a functionally naturalistic manner. Our focus in developing guidelines for each component of the DMP has been influenced by the sequences with which these decisions are actually made in designing an augmentative intervention program.

Figure 1 is a graphic illustration of these component sequences. Although they are highly interrelated (i.e., each influences the other), they clearly evolve in a sequential order. As in vocal intervention programming, evaluation procedures form the basis for all subsequent decisions. Our initial decision to augment a nonspeaker's oral speech production with a nonspeech mode (election) is followed by the selection of the specific technique to be used: static/aided, dynamic/unaided, or a combination technique. An unaided technique necessitates a dynamic system, whereas an aided technique restricts our symbol set to

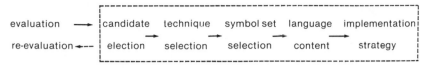

Figure 1.   Suggested components in decision making process.

a graphic system (Table 1). The constraints of a particular system will influence the form, content, and organization of the lexicon selected, and the suggested lexicon will guide the strategies selected both to teach and to use these forms efficiently. Although the sequential organization of the DMP has been described, continuous feedback flow between the components allows our later decisions to influence or revise earlier ones.

The importance of evaluation and reevaluation throughout the DMP cannot be overemphasized. It is, perhaps, useful to think of our decisions in relation to Wiener's (1948) cybernetic principles. Our decisions are actually controlled by our clients' performances rather than by the performance level we expect. By continually reevaluating our decisions in terms of *client performance and changing needs*, we can adjust our input to maximize system functioning.

As indicated above, the development of guidelines for each component in the DMP has paralleled the sequences of these decisions themselves. Some measure of sophistication has been established for evaluation, election, technique, and symbol system selection procedures. Our next natural focus (and the focus of this chapter) reflects our own clinical judgments concerning the lexical content of our intervention program.

WHAT DO WE MEAN BY LEXICAL CONTENT DECISIONS?

Imagine that you have been asked to work with a nonspeaking child. Your client is 6 years old and is cognitively functioning in the early preoperational period of development (Piaget, 1952). His comprehension skills are roughly commensurate with his cognitive abilities, and interactionally he is functionally relating at a 3 year-old level. He is ambulatory, but his gross motor and fine motor functioning are symptomatic of a left-sided hemiparesis. Because of his neuromuscular weakness, oral-motor skills are severely impaired. His "production" attempts are limited to unintelligible vocalizations and pointing. The semantic relations your client appears to code place him at phase II in the developmental sequence of language acquisition (Bloom and Lahey, 1978).

Table 1. Symbol sets and symbol systems[a]

Dynamic systems	Graphic systems	Fundamental systems
1. Idiosyncratic signal	1. Alphabet	1. Objects
2. Pantomime	Orthographic	2. Miniature objects
3. Gesture	Letters	
4. Amer-Ind	Phrases	
5. American Sign Language	Combination	
6. Manual/pedagogical systems	Phonemic	
Paget Gorman Sign System	i.t.a. (Initial Teaching Alphabet)	
Seeing Essential English	Synthesized speech	
Signing Exact English	SPEEC (Sequences of Phonemes for Efficient	
Signed English	English)	
Linguistics of Visual English	2. Logographic	
Manual English	Photographs	
7. Manual English/siglish	Pictures	
8. Total Communication	Picsyms	
9. Fingerspelling	PIC (pictogram ideogram communication)	
10. Cued speech	VIC (visual communication)	
	Blisssymbolics	
	Rhebus	
	Abstract	
	Yerkish lexigrams	
	Premack symbols	
	3. Encoding	
	Braille	
	Morse code	

[a] Adapted from McNamara (1980).

Your client has undergone a comprehensive evaluation by the interdisciplinary rehabilitation team at your facility and it has been recommended that early intervention focus on the introduction of Blissymbolics using a direct selection mode, on a manual communication board.

The initial sequences of the DMP have been completed. The child has been evaluated, the decision to "augment" has been made, an aided technique has been prescribed, and the recommended symbol set has been selected.

You are now faced with the formidable task of deciding which lexical items to teach, how to evaluate the potential usefulness of these items for your client, and how to sequence and functionally organize the introduction of this word pool. These are the lexical content decisions of your intervention program. The references listed in Table 2 were selected to aid in making such decisions.

A FUNCTIONALLY BASED NESTING MODEL

Our early lexical selection and organization decisions mirror our views concerning the application of particular models of clinical intervention. The use of a developmental model (i.e., basing intervention on the content and sequences of language acquisition and communication development in speaking children) has significantly affected our clinical methods in treating *vocal* language impaired children. Our knowledge about how children use language to reflect their ideas about the world has sensitized us to their perspectives in developing communicative skills. The identification of invariant sequences of language acquisition (Bloom and Lahey, 1978) has provided us with a viable framework with which to assess competency and target goals for intervention.

It has been asked whether atypically developing children acquire knowledge about the world in a fashion similar to normal children. Miller and Yoder (1974) have suggested that *vocal* mentally retarded children develop language in a sequence similar to that of normal children, but their development proceeds at a much slower rate. They suggested basing language intervention on the semantic notions and relations expressed by normally developing children at similar developmental levels.

Harris and Vanderheiden (1980a) have stressed that *nonvocal* techniques are not a direct substitute for *vocal* speech and that skills acquired in a seemingly invariant fashion for *vocal* nonhandicapped children may be learned through different processes and in a different order by nonspeaking severely handicapped children. Clearly we cannot assume that an atypically developing individual necessarily follows the

Table 2. Selected references for constructing an initial lexicon

Reference	Target population	Output mode	Technique	Symbol system	Augmented
Miller and Yoder, 1974	Mentally retarded children	Vocal	Unaided	Spoken words	No
Vicker, 1974	Severely physically handicapped children	Nonvocal	Aided	Graphic pictures, letters, or words	Yes
Holland, 1975	Language impaired children	Vocal	Unaided	Spoken words	No
Lahey and Bloom, 1977	Language impaired children	Vocal	Unaided	Spoken words	No
Fristoe and Lloyd, 1980	Mentally retarded and autistic individuals	Nonvocal	Unaided	Manual signs	Yes
Sailor et al., 1980	Severely and profoundly handicapped individuals	Vocal/nonvocal	Unaided/aided	Unspecified	No/yes
Wilson, 1980	Nonspeaking individuals	Nonvocal	Aided	Blissymbols/Rebus	Yes
Riechle, Williams, and Ryan, 1981	Severely handicapped individuals	Nonvocal	Unaided	Manual signs	Yes
Carlson, 1981	Nonspeaking children	Nonvocal	Unspecified	Unspecified	Yes
Perlich, 1981	Severely physically handicapped children	Nonvocal	Aided	Blisssymbols	Yes
Musselwhite and St. Louis, 1982	Severely handicapped individuals	Vocal/nonvocal	Unaided/aided	All	No/yes

same sequence of interactional, conceptual, and linguistic development shown by typically developing individuals. The nonspeaker's unique experiences may preclude strict adherence to a developmental approach to intervention.

A modification of the developmental model has been suggested by Guess, Sailor, and Baer (1977). In their remedial model, acquisition sequences commonly found in severely retarded individuals are incorporated into intervention techniques used with other similarly retarded individuals. Although the practical utility of a remedial model of this type seems plausible, our knowledge of potential similarities among members of any particular etiological group is extremely limited.

Another approach toward intervention is represented by the availability of intervention manuals containing preselected lexicons for use with nonspeaking people. The content of these programs ranges from a compilation of items clinicians have found useful for their nonspeaking clients to direct applications of psycholinguistic research reflecting the most commonly used words in the initial lexicons of developing children. "Nonspeaking" individuals are very different from one another. This variability is reflected both by the range of etiological groups from which potential candidates are selected (Table 3), and by the individual variability factors influencing the perspective of an individual client at any point in his development. Many nonspeakers have never acquired functional speech, whereas others had previously ac-

Table 3.   Potential population

Cerebral palsy
Mental retardation
Autism
Neuromuscular weakness
Oral apraxia
Aphasia
Hearing impairment
Glossectomy
Cerebral insult
Multiple sclerosis
Amyotrophic lateral sclerosis (ALS)
Parkinson's disease
Sickle cell anemia
Deaf/blind
Degenerative disease
Trauma
Multiple handicap
Emotional disorder
Other

quired speech but have permanently or temporarily lost their functional oral skills. Some have developed complex idiosyncratic signals to regulate actively their lives, whereas others have assumed a passive communicative role. In applying augmentative communication systems to such a varied group of individuals, teaching an invariant group of preselected items would hardly seem reasonable.

Additional considerations in initial lexicon selection involve constraints of the particular symbol system. Systems based on visual and tactile fingerspelling or alphabetic writing, are parasitic; that is, they simply transpose the units of speech into another modality (Studdert-Kennedy, 1980). Certain manual systems, such as American Sign Language (ASL), do not directly correspond to the words of spoken American English, nor do their rules for syntactic combination correspond to the syntax of spoken languages.

Linguistic signals do not share representational properties with their referents; the sounds and words that are conventionally used to represent objects or concepts are abstractly related to those objects and concepts. Symbol systems and manual systems vary in iconicity. Functional signs or pictographic symbols look like the objects or actions they represent. As is discussed later, the degree of iconicity of a particular item may affect ease of learning and intelligibility, which may influence the selection of particular items. Similarly, it has been suggested (Lahey and Bloom, 1977) that abstract concepts, which are difficult to demonstrate in context, may not be useful in initial lexicon planning. Although this point is well taken for vocal system intervention, abstract concepts are occasionally more easily learned in a nonvocal system. The inner state reflected by the item *want* may more easily be recognized through the manual movements symbolizing the sign than by the abstract linguistic symbols that represent its equivalent in spoken language.

Selecting an initial lexicon in augmentative communication intervention is not an easy task. There is no single intervention model that can reflect adequately the needs of the variety of nonspeaking people we will be working with. Yet, the initial lexical items that are selected are extremely important to both the nonspeaker and his family. The extent to which those items will refine the nonspeaker's ability to actively control his life and more successfully share interpersonally with others, will form the foundation and motivation for future active system use.

The approach toward intervention that may most closely reflect this notion is the use of a functionally based nesting model (Figure 2). In nested designs the embedded components cannot be viewed in isolation from the larger components that surround them. Developmental

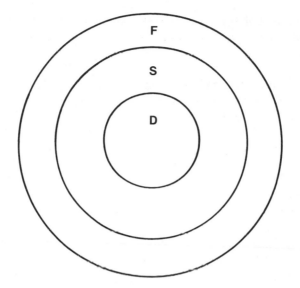

Figure 2.   A functionally based nesting model: F = functional utility, S = system constraints, D = developmental data.

data (from typical or atypical individuals) often provide invaluable guidelines for lexical selection and organization, but such data cannot be viewed separately from the constraints of the symbol system being used. An even stronger statement, however, is suggested by the proposed model. Lexical selections based on developmental guidelines and symbol system constraints must *always* be evaluated in terms of their functional usefulness for the nonspeaker.

Our primary goal in early lexicon planning is to select items that might have the *broadest functional utility* and *highest interest value* for the nonspeaker. In a functional model, lexical selection is based on the individual's unique experiences and capabilities in communicatively regulating his environment. Although we attempt to select items with the greatest potential for unassisted later language learning (Holland, 1975), our immediate goal is to identify the functions that are perceived by the nonspeaker himself, his primary caregivers, and the clinicians, to be of primary importance in promoting the nonspeaker's *immediate active* participation in controlling his own life. This core lexicon might best consist of a balance of preselected and spontaneously selected items reflecting the nonspeaker's unique interests, needs, and regularities in his daily life.

To develop this initial lexicon adequately, we must be familiar with the components of language development and communicative competency, the selected symbol system and the constraints on its use, and most important, the functional needs and capabilities of the individual who will be communicating via the lexicon we develop.

This chapter suggests a series of questions that clinicians might ask themselves in preparing this initial lexicon. The term "initial lexicon" is this context refers to the first words expressed by a nonspeaker in the early stages of language learning and/or the first words expressed by a linguistically advanced nonspeaker possessing no intelligible means of expression. The reader is advised to keep these distinctions in mind when evaluating the proposed guidelines in working with an individual nonspeaker. The questions proposed are neither disorder specific nor system specific. Their ultimate value in the design of a functionally appropriate lexicon is subject to your own clinical intuitions concerning the needs of the nonspeaker you are assisting.

INVENTORY FOR BASIC WORD POOL

In preparing a potential word pool, it is helpful to record the contexts within which each word has been identified. These contexts provide the most naturalistic settings for introducing the corresponding lexical items to the nonspeaker.

1. *Which vocabulary items might the nonspeaker consider primary?* The extent to which an individual might actively participate in developing the lexical content of his own communication system should be respected. Active participation might range from a severely retarded individual's preoccupation with a particular object to the active indication of words that are critical to the functioning of a patient with amyotrophic lateral sclerosis (ALS). Although intervention should not be restricted to those items, the nonspeaker's selections should receive high priority in constructing an initial word pool. Additionally, when treating a client with metalinguistic skills, it is important to discuss preselected items *with him* for his evaluation of their importance.

2. *Which vocabulary items do the primary caregivers stress as important?* In this context "primary caregivers" refers to the individuals who routinely interact with the nonspeaker and whose interpersonal interactions with him provide the primary treatment contexts. Frequently, primary caregivers suggest lexical items reflecting objects, events, or people of importance to the nonspeaker (the designation and training of primary caregivers as "cataloguers" has been discussed by Carlson, 1981). Related professionals may suggest items essential to the implementation of their treatment programs. The author has found recommendations from oc-

cupational therapists, physical therapists, and educators to be invaluable. Occasionally the suggested items might seem to reflect the needs of the primary caregiver instead of the nonspeaker. A mother might say, "If only he could tell me he's hungry," or "If he could just say 'Mama.'" If we accept the viewpoints that a significant aspect of language development is its interpersonal function and that sensitivity to both participants is crucial to communicative interaction development, we will respect these requests and include these items in our word pool inventory.

3. *Which items reflect routine events experienced by the nonspeaker?* In many respects our lives are organized by routines. We wake up at a specified time, hop into the shower, slip on our clothes, down two cups of coffee, and catch the 7:45 express to the clinic. These actions represent routine events in our daily lives. Nonspeakers' lives are similarly routinized. Clinical experience suggests that many handicapped people experience rigid routines throughout the day. Severely to profoundly handicapped children in a residential setting may have little variety in their daily schedules. Sequences of events or scripts, as defined in the cognitive literature (e.g., Nelson, 1981; Rifkin, 1981), provide a rich source of lexical items for the initial word pool inventory. Although it has been suggested that rigid routines promote passivity and inhibit initiatory communication attempts for the nonspeaker, clinical experience suggests that selection of lexical items reflective of these events and introduction of these items within the naturalistic contexts of the actual events are highly successful in developing communicative interaction skills for multiply handicapped nonspeakers. Additionally, by occasionally breaching the sequences of a routine, and by providing the nonspeaker with the lexicon to select preferred items within the routine, initiation skills in conversation are often stimulated.

4. *Which items reflect preferences or dislikes for objects, actions, or people in the environment?* This question suggests the selection of lexical terms representing items of high interest value for the nonspeaker. High interest value has generally meant preferred objects, people, and events in the nonspeaker's life. The author's clinical experience suggests expanding "high interest value" to include objects, people, and events that are strongly disliked by the nonspeaker. A prime motivational factor in communicative interaction is our ability to exert some degree of control over the occurrences in our lives. This regulation reflects not only our successful obtainment of preferred items but also our ability to reject interaction with particular items. This factor may strongly influence the non-

speaker's realization that communicative interaction can have naturally rewarding consequences. As suggested by Holland (1975), we are teaching our clients that language is used for more than obtaining a token or candy—rather, they are experiencing the naturally rewarding consequences of being understood, being granted a request, and so on.

5. *Which words reflect basic bodily needs and internal/emotional states?* This guideline is probably the most frequently used suggestion in traditional intervention programs. Communicative interaction focuses around more than fulfillment of basic needs, yet items reflecting these needs are important sources for the initial word pool inventory. Basic needs are precisely that: basic to an individual's functioning. If a person is hungry, angry, or in pain, it's unlikely that he will be free to communicate about anything else. Although the cognitive level of the nonspeaker influences the inclusion of particular items reflecting internal states, often expletives or exclamations can be used by a nonspeaker who may not be ready to discuss his internal feelings. Terms such as "Yay!", "Oh boy," and "xxxxxx" (frustration expletive) are spontaneous expressions of joy or anger. When we are disappointed or furious we often blurt out an expletive before we can clearly articulate our feelings. The nonspeaker's initial lexicon should have optimal value for the spontaneous expression of feelings while simultaneously enabling the listener to interpret those states.

6. *Which communicative functions and semantic notions are currently being expressed by the nonspeaker through residual oral speech and idiosyncratic signal systems? Which items might code these functions?* Suggested here is the systematic analysis of how the nonspeaker is currently using his communication system in interacting and attempting to identify his knowledge of the world in terms of the meaningful relations and interpersonal functions he "naturally" expresses. Items that can enhance his skills in communicating these functional relations provide a rich source for the basic word pool inventory. This question also emphasizes our need to devise an intervention program based on what an individual can do (i.e., client performance) instead of what we expect or would like him to do.

7. *Which lexical items do you intuitively feel might have maximal functional value for the nonspeaker?* Although the systematic consideration of the foregoing questions should yield a sizable preliminary word pool, usually additional items are suggested by your personal relationship with the nonspeaker. There may be notions that you feel the nonspeaker might productively express, given the

means to express them, items not yet included that are highly useful for a nonspeaker (e.g., to gain attention, to express affirmation/negation), or items directly reflective of your personal relationship with the nonspeaker (*us* words). All items should be reevaluated in terms of their functional utility and interest value for the nonspeaker, and words reflecting your own clinical intuitions should be included in the preliminary word pool inventory.

SYSTEM CONSTRAINTS

Fristoe and Lloyd (1980) have stressed the importance of our familiarity with manual signs and the constraints on their use as a prerequisite feature in planning an initial expressive sign lexicon. This fact holds true for any symbol system we are using with our nonspeaking clients. In compiling the word pool inventory, we have attempted to identify items that are relevant to the nonspeaker's daily life. Those items, however, reflect the auditory vocal mode with which most of us communicate our ideas about the world. Our next task is to "translate" those meanings into the corresponding modality of the symbol system that has been selected. These forms can then be examined to assess their suitability for a particular client.

1. *How transparent or iconic is the symbol?* Symbol sets, such as manual signs or logographic systems, can be described in terms of their iconicity. Klima and Bellugi (1979) have defined iconicity as the degree to which the elements of a sign or symbol are related to visual aspects of what is denoted. Despite a paucity of support for the notion that the meaning of iconic signs can be readily guessed by a nonsigner, there has been evidence (Nietupski and Hamre-Nietupski, 1979) that iconic signs are more easily learned than signs that are nonrepresentational. Riechle, Williams, and Ryan (1981) have divided iconicity into functional and representational classes. The topology of functional iconic signs is identical to the action produced in the activity represented by the sign (e.g., "drink"). Representational iconic signs also show the action associated with an activity, but the topography is not identical to the action (e.g., "walk").

   It is often useful to divide signs and symbols that express degrees of iconicity on three representational levels. Signs can be evaluated in terms of their transparency (clear relation to the appearance or action of the object or event), translucency (representational relation to the object or action), and opaqueness (abstract relationship of sign and referent).

Similarly, Blissymbolics, a meaning based logographic communication system, is divisible into three levels of iconicity: pictographic (in which a symbol looks like its referent), ideographic (in which the symbol represents an idea about the action or object), and arbitrary (reflecting the abstract relation of sign and referent). The examples in Figure 3 illustrate the range of iconicity just described.

The level of symbol or sign iconicity may not influence the utility of an item for some nonspeaking individuals. For other nonspeakers (e.g., clients with severe cognitive impairment or young children), it may strongly influence both rate and ease of learning. The author recommends evaluating the items selected for the initial word pool in terms of their iconicity. The clients' individual strengths and weaknesses will influence the selection procedures.

2.   *How easily can an item be produced by an individual?* The physical or motor characteristics of signs (the use of one hand or two handed signs, hands performing identical or nonidentical movements, etc.) have various effects on the ease with which signs may be produced or learned by particular clients. In assessing the appropriateness of teaching a lexical item, it can be useful to evaluate the selected signs in terms of these characteristics in relation to the skills of the nonspeaker. Based on Piaget's view that initially learners are

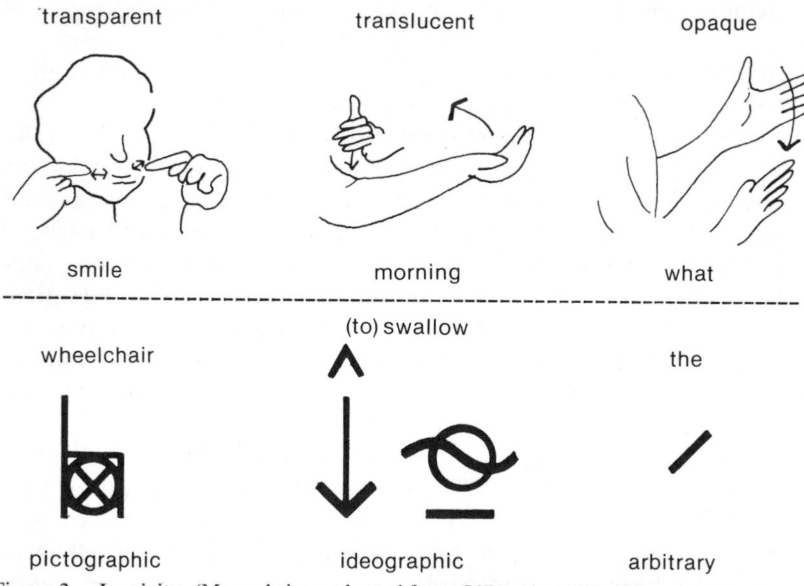

Figure 3.   Iconicity. (Manual signs adapted from O'Rourke, 1973. Blissymbolics © used herein. Blissymbolics Communication Institute, 1982, Toronto, Canada.)

best able to imitate behaviors already within their repertoire, Riechle et al. (1981) have suggested the potential relevance of selecting in-repertoire behaviors in the selection of initial signs. Clinical experience supports the notion that signs that are comprised of physical movements the nonspeaker is already using and, additionally, may be clearly visible to him, may affect ease of learning, as well as the ability to place these movements under contingency control. Although ease of production varies with the skills of the individual nonspeaker, it is not useful to rule out automatically a particular item because of the complexity of the movements. Occasionally an item that seems to be complex might be produced skillfully by the nonspeaker. As discussed earlier, our decisions should reflect actual client performance, not the performance we expect of them. Thus in familiarizing ourselves with these constraints, and in rating the selected lexicon for this complexity, we should be able to make clinically sound judgments for the selection of the lexicon.

3. *How perceptually complex is the symbol?* Lexical items should be evaluated in terms of their perceptual complexity. Figure 4a illustrates this feature. The sign for "forever" begins with the index finger moving away from the face in a semicircular motion; it then loops into a counterclockwise circular motion, terminating in a y-hand glide away from the body. By producing this sign in front of a mirror, perceptual complexity can be clearly identified. Similarly the Blissymbolic for "clothing" entails a complex figure-ground component. The degree to which perceptual complexity will affect the nonspeaker's recognition and productive use of an item might be considered in selection decisions.

4. *How topographically similar are the items being introduced?* Items sharing physical or natural features are frequently confused. Signs and symbols are similar to sounds to the extent to which each can be described in terms of a set of distinctive features. Signs can be described in terms of movement, handshape configuration, place of articulation, and orientation, whereas symbols (e.g., Blissymbolics) may be defined by their shape, position, spacing, direction, and size. Items that differ in one distinctive feature may be more difficult to discriminate than items differing in two or more features. Examples of signs and symbols sharing physically similar features are illustrated in Figure 4b. The signs for "children" and "things" are identical in handshape, place of articulation, and movement, but differ in palm orientation. Similarly, the Blissymbolics for "happy" and "sad" share all but one feature, the direction of the pointer. Clinical experience suggests that for some

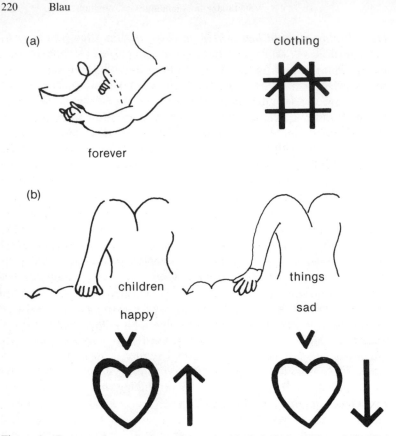

(a) clothing

forever

(b)

children

things

happy

sad

Figure 4.   Perceptual complexity and topographical similarity. (Manual signs adapted from O'Rourke, 1973. Blissymbolics © used herein, Blissymbolics Communications Institute, 1982, Toronto, Canada.

nonspeakers it may be advisable to reduce the number of topographically similar items in developing an initial lexicon. The inclusion of certain items may be postponed, or compensatory strategies designed, to avoid item confusion.

Another type of confusion that is not physical but meaning based that occasionally occurs between items of an event class. Distinctions between items of clothing (shoes and socks) or eating utensils (fork, knife, and spoon), although not physically related, have an association with the event or object class they represent. A nonspeaker may have no difficulty in learning the appropriate items, but clinical experience indicates that some nonspeakers experience a great deal of confusion when using these related lexical items.

5. *How intelligibly and how efficiently can the item be produced by the nonspeaker?* This question is representative of the information we obtain through trial teaching. Children learning language do not necessarily produce accurate replications of adult words until they have progressed well beyond the early stages of language acquisition. Similarly, we should not expect perfection from the nonspeaker, whether he is a developmentally delayed child or a cognitively mature adult. A clear illustration of this principle is the range of abilities displayed by the staff members at any treatment facility when learning symbol systems. The first items used by a nonspeaker greatly influence his realization of the communicative value for using his symbol set; therefore the degree to which listeners can interpret the selected item should be part of the DMP.

6. *How clearly do photographs, pictures, or small objects reflect the salient properties of the object or event being introduced?* It is important to keep in mind the individual nonspeaker's perspective in trying to determine what he might see as salient. In our selection of photos, pictures, and objects, we have predetermined knowledge (presuppositional knowledge) of what the items will be representing. How clearly do those items reflect the nonspeaker's knowledge of the world?

EVALUATION OF SELECTED ITEMS

An initial lexicon should include a small number of dynamically useful items, as opposed to a large static vocabulary pool. Examination of each item in terms of the selected symbol set modality will consolidate the original word pool. We might next attempt to refine and sequence our selections by evaluating each item in terms of its functional utility and interest value for the nonspeaker.

1. *Which of the selected items may be used to code a variety of communicative functions?* It has been suggested (e.g., Greenfield and Smith, 1976; Harris and Vanderheiden, 1980a; Slobin, 1973) that children first learning to talk code one word for one function. As their language skills develop, they begin to use the same words to express a variety of functions. For example, children may initially produce the word "ball" to code existence, as a labeling function, during a familiar play routine with Mom. Later on, they might express "ball" to request the ball, to comment that they have a ball, to get Mother to look at the ball, to indicate that the ball has fallen or is gone, or perhaps to greet the ball. Items that

can potentially code the variety of communicative functions or semantic notions a child is currently expressing or might express possess a high degree of functional utility. Similarly adults or children who are restricted by the number of items available to them because of the spatial limitations of an augmentative technique will find greater value in items that can code a wide range of communicative functions.

2. *Which items have potential use for multiword combinations?* Holland's (1975) organization of a sample core lexicon for language impaired children stresses its maximal potential for serving as a basis for later unassisted language growth and use. The selected items might be combined to express a variety of grammatical functions. Lahey and Bloom's (1977) organization of lexical items according to content categories similarly reflects the items' potential growth into two-word utterances. Our own evaluation of the items we have selected in terms of the various multiword combinations that are functionally usable for the nonspeaker, will promote optimal use of the lexicon.

The constraints of the selected symbol set will additionally provide guidelines concerning items highly useful for multiword combinations. Symbol systems, such as Amerind (Skelly, 1979) and Blissymbolics (Silverman, McNaughton, and Kates, 1978), reflect the principle of agglutination, in which earlier learned gestures and shapes are combined to produce more complex gestures and new forms. Core lexical items, which can be agglutinated, will be high in functional utility for the nonspeaker.

3. *Which items can best reflect the "here and now"? Which reflect preferences for objects, people, and events not salient in the immediate context?* A recurrent theme in the literature has been the importance of the "here and now" in children's talk and the stimulation of language in context. Children, in the early stages of language learning, talk about what they are doing or are about to do. Items should be evaluated for usefulness in expressing ongoing events. Although it is important to introduce these items in context, we might also consider the unique needs of the nonspeaker. Adult and cognitively mature nonspeakers often prefer lexical items representing people, objects, and events that are unavailable in the immediate context. Severely physically handicapped individuals are less able to act on their environments and may speak less of what they are doing and more of what they have done or are expecting to do. Nonspeakers are often the recipients of a barrage of questions. These questions rarely ask "What are you doing now?" but more frequently inquire "What

did you do last week?'' or ''What will you be doing next week?''
Attempting to enrich the nonspeaker's ability to act on the world
and talk about these actions is desirable, but we should also recognize the realistic features that comprise the nonspeaker's life
and select items that best reflect this reality.

4. *Which items can the nonspeaker express using residual oral, non-
    verbal, or idiosyncratic signaling systems?* This question reflects
    a deeper concern: Do we select items the individual can presently
    communicate with his idiosyncratic signal system? As with all the
    considerations presented thus far, the answer to this question
    depends on the individual nonspeaker. Our goal in developing an
    initial lexicon is not to replace with more conventional forms an
    individual's present means of interacting in the world. Rather, we
    want to enhance that existing ability. Keeping the nonspeaker's
    perspective foremost in our minds, we know that his idiosyncratic
    signals are part of his identity and have been his primary method
    for successfully controlling aspects of his life. Perhaps our initial
    focus might be on enhancing his ability to transmit more suc-
    cessfully these signals (by providing additional forms for them),
    or on teaching forms for functions he cannot transmit via his sig-
    naling system.

    We also need to be sensitive to the needs of both participants
in communicative interactions. Perhaps an individual's signals are
clear to his primary caregivers but unclear to other significant
people in his life. Perhaps the nonspeaker's lifestyle promotes
frequent interactions with nonfamiliar listeners. In selecting lexical items for each individual nonspeaker within the context of
his needs, we must focus on efficiency and effectiveness in communication.

    Speakers as well as nonspeakers use a host of cues to transmit
and interpret messages (Higginbotham and Yoder, 1982). In addition to verbal output (vocal or nonvocal), we rely on paralinguistic information (prosody) and nonverbal cues (body language)
in our communicative interactions (Table 4). The nonspeaker's
residual oral and paralinguistic skills and nonverbal expressions,
which may have been the source of his idiosyncratic signaling
system, are rich sources for increasing the communicative functions and notions expressible with a limited set of symbols. The
questioning function can often be expressed by the wrinkling of
a brow or a rise in intonation. The use of a single item, such as
''understand,'' can serve as a question when accompanied by
facial expression or vocal inflection, or can serve as a back-channel response (similar to ''Oh, I see'') when accompanied by a

Table 4. Cues used to transmit
and interpret messages[a]

Verbal (vocal/nonvocal)
   Spoken word
   Written word
   Manual sign
   Graphic symbol
Paralinguistic
   Intonation contour
   Pitch
   Vocal quality
   Melody
   Intensity
   Extent
   Prosodic features
Nonverbal
   Body posture
   Body orientation
   Muscular tension
   Hand movements
   Facial expressions
   Eye gaze
   Distance between participants
   Physical contact

[a] This description of the complex
and highly interrelated features of the
human communication system has been
oversimplified for the sake of brevity.

head nod. We should evaluate the idiosyncratic signals of our
nonspeaking clients in the contexts of their functional abilities
and make maximum use of such symbols in planning an initial
lexicon.

5. *How frequently might the item be used in a particular setting or
in a variety of settings?* Items that can be frequently used throughout the nonspeaker's day will hold high functional value and will
provide numerous contexts for learning. It has been suggested
that teaching novel situations to express existing communicative
functions should come after an individual is competently using
that item within familiar contexts; words having high generaliz-
ability across situations, however, can maximally promote language use. Riechle et al. (1981) have emphasized that frequency
of vocabulary use should be determined by the nonspeaker's
wants and needs as opposed to frequency of use by speaking
individuals.

6. *How much information can be conveyed by the symbol?* Certain
lexical items are holophrastic; that is, the expression of a single

item serves to convey a complete proposition. The greater the amount of information that can be clearly transmitted to the listener with a limited set of items, the more useful those items will be for the nonspeaker.

7. *How high in reinforcement value is the symbol for the nonspeaker?* The key phrase used here is "for the individual." To evaluate the potential reinforcement value of an item, the clinician must make this judgment with the likes and dislikes of the individual in mind. Items that are reinforcing to one person may not be reinforcing to another. A word that clearly transmits the nonspeaker's intention to a listener will generally hold high reinforcement value and its use will increase.

Sailor et al. (1980), in discussing initial responses of severely retarded individuals, suggested that although high frequency of occurrence is crucial, an item with intrinsically reinforcing properties, even if used less frequently, may have a greater potential for use. For example, severely handicapped students may frequently experience being buckled in and out of their wheelchairs, and "seatbelt" may not be a particularly reinforcing item. "Brush," however, used in the context of hairbrushing, may be a less frequently used object but nevertheless particularly reinforcing to a child. Additionally, the authors suggested that items that provide sensory feedback (music, bell, light) may be highly reinforcing to children. These items may not represent frequently occurring activities in the child's natural environment, but they rely on natural, response specific, powerful reinforcers and are potentially useful in teaching initial communicative responses. The author's experience in working with multiply handicapped children supports this notion; however, caution should be used in providing indiscriminate sensory stimulation to a tactilely defensive cerebral palsy child or light emitting reinforcers to an individual who is prone to seizures.

8. *How much nonlinguistic support is available for introducing the item? How easily can the concept be demonstrated in context?* Lahey and Bloom (1977) stress the importance of two related factors—availability of nonlinguistic support and ease of demonstrating a concept in context—in selecting initial lexical items for language impaired children. These factors are equally important in the selection of lexical items for nonspeaking individuals. The amount of nonlinguistic support needed to introduce a particular item will reflect the cognitive level of the nonspeaker and the form of his experience with the object or event. Items reflecting an individual's active experiences may be learned more

easily than items reflecting passive experiences. Lahey and Bloom have suggested that concepts that are difficult to demonstrate in context should be presented after items more readily illustrated in context. In working with cognitively and linguistically mature nonspeakers, this suggestion may be less critical. However, we should try to select items that reflect concepts or properties that are clearly salient to the nonspeaking individual.

9. *Which items can potentially be used in peer interaction and play?* Lexical items that are functionally useful in interacting with peers will enrich both utility and interest value for the nonspeaker. Clinical experience suggests that highly iconic items are more easily retained by the nonspeaker's peers. Selecting functionally useful items that are also part of the nonspeaking peers' lexicon provides excellent opportunities for interpersonal sharing.

Miller and Yoder (1974) have suggested that imaginative and representational play, in combination with appropriate stimulation within living environments, forms an important foundation for cognitive and linguistic development. For a nonspeaking physically handicapped child, play may be limited to activating simple battery operated toys, or, in some cases, directing someone through lexical use. Items that can promote creative play will have high motivational and educational content for the nonspeaker.

For adolescents and adults, items useful for social encounters with peers are extremely important. By selecting lexical items that enable a nonspeaker to ask a friend out on a date or tell a joke to make a friend smile will reflect the clinician's sensitivity to the social needs of the nonspeaker.

10. *Have we included polar opposites of lexical items?* Polar opposites refer to antonym pairs of words (primarily adjectives). Items such as "happy/sad," "big/little," and "hot/cold," reflect contrasts of related concepts. Lahey and Bloom (1977) have suggested that teaching polar opposites at the same time can be confusing to a child. Additionally, since the contrasts can be expressed by negation and attribution ("not happy"), postponing the teaching of these contrasts was also suggested by Lahey and Bloom. Similarly, Fristoe and Lloyd (1980) recommended postponing the inclusion of marked members of polar opposites in the initial expressive sign lexicon of mentally retarded and autistic children.

This suggestion may be advisable when using logographic symbol sets, such as Blissymbolics. The symbol for "sad" (Figure 4b) can be represented by negation plus the symbol for "happy" or by the use of the strategy marker for "opposite" plus the symbol "happy." This strategy may be maximally beneficial when paired items share topographically similar features, and may additionally stimulate the spontaneous use of multiword combinations.

We might also consider, however, that the exclusion of a particular polar opposite might not be functional for a nonspeaker who has difficulty combining items or has frequent need for each item of the pair. Generally, pairs of items frequently used or directly related to basic bodily needs should be included.

11. *Have we included items coding affirmation and negation?* The inclusion of "no," as evidenced above, is functionally useful in an initial lexicon. "No" can be used to code a variety of reflexive relations and can readily be combined with both relational and substantive words in multiword combinations.

If the nonspeaker has a clearly interpretable "no" signal, the inclusion of an additional "no" symbol might be postponed. Clinical experience suggests that nonspeakers will use their natural idiosyncratic signals to convey negation more readily than the symbols placed on their communication boards. It is important, however, to use a variety of modes to teach this important item, to ensure the nonspeaker's successful communication of his intentions to both familiar and nonfamiliar listeners.

The item "yes" also has enormous utility in augmentative communication. Constrained by nonfunctional oral skills and often by severe physical limitations, the nonspeaker lives in a world of yes/no questions. Often, the degree to which he can exert some control over his life depends on the intelligibility and efficiency of his yes/no responses.

Although it has been suggested frequently that the nonspeaker's ability to express negation and affirmation is an important prerequisite for augmentative communication intervention, it is the opinion of the author that it is not a necessary condition for *beginning* augmentative intervention. Children begin communicatively interacting before they can respond to yes/no questions. Delaying the introduction of a lexicon until a consistent yes/no is exhibited is not suggested in early augmentative programming.

12. *Have we included items for colors and body parts?* The inclusion of colors in language intervention programming has been the subject of recent debate. The communicative value of teaching attributes of color has been questioned because it has been pointed out that adults rarely label colors unless contrasting two identical objects. Lahey and Bloom (1977) have reported that the use of color attribution is not found in children's early language productions.

The communicative value of identifying colors may be questioned, but for some nonspeakers the inclusion of items chosen to indicate colors is extremely useful. If an individual is attempting to request an object for which he has no symbol and because of physical limitations cannot directly retrieve the item for himself, identification of an item by color combined with eye pointing can significantly improve communication. Additionally, symbols placed on a communication board are often categorized by color, and many encoding techniques that are used to compensate for spatial and physical limitations depend on the nonspeaker's ability to identify colors.

Perlich (1981) has commented on the absence from lexicons of items representing body parts. Body part identification routines are frequently part of a child's earliest interpersonal play and communicative turn taking experiences. Perlich has suggested that the frequency with which mother's partake in body part routines reflects the importance of these routines. Additionally, in symbol systems such as Blissymbolics, the symbols for basic body parts (mouth, ear, nose, etc.) provide the basic shapes for the complex symbols that are used to code actions and objects. It has been Perlich's clinical experience that many nonspeakers easily move from indicating symbols for body parts to indicating verbs agglutinated from body parts.

13. *How much interest value might the item hold for the nonspeaker at the time it is being introduced?* The importance of this question cannot be overemphasized. Although we are attempting to select and organize an initial lexicon in terms of its functional utility for the nonspeaker, we must also keep in mind the interest value of the selected items. Interest value reflects more than the objects, people, and events of importance to an individual. Interest value should be high when we are *introducing* an item to the nonspeaker. This consideration, again, reflects our continuous sensitivity to the nonspeaker's perspective. His interests are the foundation for the functional utility of the items we select. Additionally, if an item that we have not preselected for or with the nonspeaker is nevertheless interesting to him, we should teach that item within its natural context. Communicative interaction is a dynamic and creative exchange between partners in dialogue and it is important that we remain flexible in our programming. It is common for children and adults to use particular words and then abandon them for a while as experiences, interest, and environments change. If we are spatially limited in the amount of items we can include on a communication board, items that are no longer being used by the nonspeaker can temporarily be eliminated, and items of immediate interest substituted. (Carlson,

1981, has reached the same conclusion.) We are attempting to reinforce the nonspeaker's notions that we are helping him to build *his* communication system, that he has the choice of accepting or rejecting our suggestions, and that in using his initial lexicon he can potentially experience greater control over the occurrences in his life.

DIALOGUE IN DISCOURSE

The primary focus of this chapter is on the selection and organization of an initial lexicon for nonspeaking individuals. It is also beneficial, however, to discuss these lexical items as important features of discourse.

As discussed by Rees (1978), communicative competency reflects more than the speaker's construction of semantically, syntactically, and pragmatically intact utterances. Discourse implies the dyad. The success with which an utterance is transmitted depends on both the speaker's ability to express himself and the listener's ability to interpret what is said. Equally important is the speaker's skill in monitoring the listener for comprehension of the messages transmitted. Communicative interaction involves sharing, turn taking, and giving a response when required. In their early communicative attempts, children often focus on "the centrality of 'me'" (Holland 1975, p. 517). Their early attempts at conveying needs are expressed as minicommands, but as they mature, their mothers socialize them to the appropriate ways of using language communicatively. They learn principles of politeness (Lakoff, 1973) as well as the cooperative principle, as defined by Grice (1975). Without sensitivity to the listener, meaning cannot easily be shared. Children learn to rely on listener's verbal and nonverbal expressions to judge the success with which their messages are transmitted, and they learn techniques for initiating topics, requesting clarification, and providing back-channel responses to speakers when *they* assume the role of listener. They learn the "prospective/retrospective" approach to discourse—that is, they must often wait for a stretch of discourse to be completed before they fully understand the impact of a particular utterance (Garfinkel, 1967). Nonspeaking individuals similarly need to learn these rules of discourse. The selection of lexical items for the nonspeaker's initial lexicon should include items that promote coherently flowing exchanges between themselves and their listeners.

When nonspeaking individuals begin using language they are often unaware of the features of discourse that promote effective interaction. Frequently nonspeakers are not aware of, or may not have the lexical items for, being polite or signaling their desire to change topics or terminate the conversation. Expressions that convey these functions can be included in lexicon planning. Table 5 lists examples of social organization devices that might be included in initial lexicon planning.

A particular discourse feature the author has found to be exceedingly important, but rarely included in intervention programs, is the use of back-channel responses (Duncan, 1975; Yngve, 1970). Back channels are feedback responses that listeners give speakers to indicate that the message is being received and that the speaker may continue talking. Speakers, in turn, look for these back channels to determine whether their messages are being understood and agreed with (Table 5). A frequent source of communication breakdown between speaking and nonspeaking people is the speaker's underestimation of the nonspeaker's cognitive status. As the speaker conveys his ideas or feelings to the nonspeaker, his gaze intermittently focuses on the nonspeaker for feedback regarding the successful transmission of his message. A typical occurrence in dyadic interaction between speaking and nonspeaking individuals is the lack or absence of back channels signaled by the nonspeaker. The speaker then assumes that his message has not been transmitted and that the nonspeaker either does not understand or is uninterested, and he subsequently simplifies his speech or terminates the conversation.

It is not enough for us to teach speaking people to be sensitive to the needs of nonspeakers. We also need to stress to nonspeakers the

Table 5.   Social organization devices[a]

Boundary markers, indicating openings, closings, changes in topic
Hi
Bye
By the way
But
Also
Politeness markers, indicating sensitivity to participant
Please
Thanks
Sorry
Excuse me
Back-channel responses, maintaining flow of conversation
Yes
Uh huh
Mm hm
OK
Head nod
Eye gaze
Smile

[a] Adapted from Dore (1978).

importance of their sensitivity to the speaking people with whom they interact. Communicative interaction is much more than a medium for basic needs fulfillment. Equally important is the fulfillment of the human need to share meaning with another person. It is through the interpersonal sharing of words through the consensus of *both* partici- pants that meaning is generated (Dore, 1983; Voloshinov, 1973).

ACKNOWLEDGMENTS

The author thanks Rivkah Blau, John Dore, Margaret Lahey, and Anthony Rifkin for their thoughtful comments on an earlier draft of this chapter.

REFERENCES

Bloom, L., and Lahey, M. 1978. Language Development and Language Dis- orders. Wiley, New York.

Carlson, F. 1981. A format for selecting vocabulary for the non-speaking child. Lang. Speech Hear. Serv. Schools 12(4):240–245.

Chapman, R. S., and Miller, J. F. 1980. Analyzing language and communi- cation in the child. In: R. L. Schiefelbusch (ed.), Nonspeech Language and Communication. University Park Press, Baltimore.

Dore, J. 1978. Requestive systems in nursery school conversations: Analysis of talk in its social context. In: R. Campbell and P. Smith (eds.), Recent Advances in the Psychology of Language: Language Development and Mother-Child Interaction. Plenum Press, New York.

Dore, J. 1983. Feeling, form, and intention in the baby's transition to language. In: R. Golinkoff (ed.), From Prelinguistic to Linguistic Communication. Lawrence Erlbaum Associates, Hillsdale, N.J.

Duncan, S. 1975. On the structure of speaker-auditor interaction during speak- ing turns. Lang. Society 2:161–180.

Fristoe, M., and Lloyd, L. 1980. Planning an initial expressive sign lexicon for persons with severe communication impairment. J. Speech Hear. Disord. 45(2):170–180.

Garfinkel, H. 1967. Studies in Ethnomethodology. Prentice-Hall, Englewood Cliffs, N.J.

Greenfield, P., and Smith, J. 1976. The Structure of Communication in Early Language Development. Academic Press, New York.

Grice, H. P. 1975. Logic and conversation. In: P. Cole and J. L. Morgan (eds.), Syntax and Semantics, Vol. 3. Speech Acts. Academic Press, New York.

Guess, D., Sailor, W., and Baer, D. 1977. A behavioral-remedial approach to language training for the severely handicapped individual. In: E. Sontag (ed.), Educational Programming for the Severely and Profoundly Handi- capped, pp. 360–377. Division on Mental Retardation, CEC, Reston, Va.

Harris, D., and Vanderheiden, G. 1980a. Enhancing the development of com- municative interaction. In: R. L. Schiefelbusch (ed.), Nonspeech Language and Communication. University Park Press, Baltimore.

Harris, D., and Vanderheiden, G. 1980b. Augmentative communication tech- niques. In: R. L. Schiefelbusch (ed.), Nonspeech Language and Commu- nication. University Park Press, Baltimore.

Higginbotham, D. J., and Yoder, D. E. 1982. Communication within natural conversational interaction: Implications for severe communicatively impaired persons. Topics Lang. Disord. 2(2):1–19.

Holland, A. 1975. Language therapy for children: Some thoughts on context and content. J. Speech Hear. Disord. 40:514–523.

Klima, E., and Bellugi, U. 1979. The Signs of Language. Harvard University Press, Cambridge, Mass.

Lahey, M., and Bloom, L. 1977. Planning a first lexicon: Which words to teach first. J. Speech Hear. Disord. 42:340–349.

Lakoff, R. 1973. The logic of politeness; or minding your p's and q's. In: C. Corum, T. Smith-Clark, and A. Weiser (eds.), Papers from the Ninth Regional Meeting of the Chicago Linguistic Society. University of Chicago Press, Chicago.

McNamara, R. D. 1980. Symbol systems in augmentative communication. Paper presented at Augmentative Communication Workshop, Goldwater Memorial Hospital, New York.

Meyers, L., Grows, N., Coleman, C., and Cook, A. 1980. An assessment battery for assistive device system recommendations, Part I. Technical Report no. 1. California State University, Sacramento.

Miller, J., and Yoder, D. 1974. An ontogenetic language training strategy for retarded children. In: R. L. Schiefelbusch and L. Lloyd (eds.), Language Perspectives: Acquisition, Retardation, and Intervention. University Park Press, Baltimore.

Musselwhite, C. R., and St. Louis, K. W. 1982. Communication Programming for the Severely Handicapped: Vocal and Non-vocal strategies. College Hill Press, Houston.

Nelson, K. 1981. Social cognition in a script framework. In: L. Ross and J. Flavell (eds.), Social Cognitive Development: Frontiers and Possible Futures. Cambridge University Press, New York.

Nietupski, J., and Hamre-Nietupski, S. 1979. Teaching auxilliary communication skills to severely handicapped students. Am. Assoc. Educ. Severely Profoundly Handicapped 4:107–124.

O'Rourke, T. J. 1973. A Basic Course in Manual Communication. National Association of the Deaf, Silver Spring, Md.

Perlich, C. 1981. Initial Blissymbol lexicons. Newsletter (Blissymbolics Communication Institute) 25:13–19.

Piaget, J. 1952. The Origins of Intelligence in Children. Norton, New York.

Rees, N. 1978. Pragmatics of language. In: R. L. Schiefelbusch (ed.), Bases of Language Intervention. University Park Press, Baltimore.

Riechle, J., Williams, W., and Ryan, S. 1981. Selecting signs for the formulation of an augmentative communication modality. J. Assoc. Severely Handicapped 6:48–56.

Rifkin, A. J. 1981. Event categories, event taxonomies, and basic level events: An initial investigation. Unpublished manuscript. Graduate School and University Center, City University of New York, New York.

Sailor, W., Guess, D., Goetz, L., Schuler, A., Utley, B., and Baldwin, M. 1980. Language and severely handicapped persons—Deciding what to teach to whom. In: W. Sailor, B. Wilcox, and L. Brown (eds.), Methods of Instruction for Severely Handicapped Students. Brookes Publishing Co., Baltimore.

Shane, H. 1981. Decision making in early augmentative communication use. In: R. L. Schiefelbusch (ed.), Early Language: Acquisition and Intervention. University Park Press, Baltimore.

Silverman, H., McNaughton, S., and Kates, B. 1978. Handbook of Blissymbolics. Blissymbolics Communication Institute, Toronto, Ont., Canada.

Skelly, M. 1979. Amer-Ind Gestural Code. Elsevier, New York.

Slobin, D. I. 1973. Cognitive prerequisites for the development of grammar. In: C. A. Ferguson and D. I. Slobin (eds.), Studies of Child Language Development. Holt, Rinehart and Winston, New York.

Studdert-Kennedy, M. 1980. The beginnings of speech. In: G. B. Barlow, K. Immelmann, M. Main, and L. Petronovich (eds.), Behavioral Development: The Bielefeld Interdisciplinary Project. Cambridge University Press, New York.

Vanderheiden, G. 1980. Selecting Appropriate Communication and Control aids: A Parallel Profile Approach. Trace Resource and Development Center. University of Wisconsin, Madison.

Vicker, B. 1974. Nonoral Communication Project 1964/1973. University of Iowa, Campus Stores Pub., Iowa City.

Voloshinov, V. N. 1973. Marxism and the Philosophy of Language. Seminar Press, New York.

Wiener, N. 1948. Cybernetics. Sci. Am. 179:14–19.

Wilson, K. D. 1980. Selection of a core lexicon for use with graphic communication systems. J. Child Commun. Disord. 4:111–123.

Yngve, V. H. 1970. On getting a word in edgewise. Papers from the Sixth Regional Meeting of the Chicago Linguistic Society. Chicago Linguistic Society, Chicago.

CHAPTER 13

Microcomputers
A Clinical Aid

Mary S. Wilson and *Bernard J. Fox*

Advances in computer technology indicate that computers can be valuable teaching tools in speech and language rehabilitation. Wilson and Fox provide a rationale for their use and describe several applications.

1. *Wilson and Fox recommend the use of computer presented material for teaching language. What kinds of material can be programmed? With what population of language delayed children is computer presented material appropriate? Do language delayed children respond well to material presented by a computer?*
2. *Describe the two feedback procedures that Wilson and Fox recommend in the presentation of language material by computer. Did they find these procedures to be effective?*
3. *Throughout the chapter Wilson and Fox indicate several reasons for using computer presented material in language training. How many reasons can you find? Do you agree with the authors?*

MICROCOMPUTERS HAVE ARRIVED. They come with cute names like Apple and Pet, but they are not toys; they are powerful machines that promise to affect our lives. Over the past year unit sales of microcomputers have accelerated. Even IBM entered the personal computer market in 1981, surely another indicator that small computers are here to stay. Indeed, current and predicted user growth curves indicate that microcomputers will become as ubiquitous by 1990 as hand-held calculators are now. You may recall that those calculators didn't exist a decade ago.

What will the microcomputer age mean for us professionally? For some time we have accepted computers as part of our research and administrative lives, but now microcomputers are moving into our homes, schools, and clinics. Over the next decade microcomputers will be playing an increasingly important role in our profession. The question no longer is will we use them in our clinical work, but how will we use them or, perhaps more important, how should we use them? Before tackling that question we should step back and look at these machines, and determine what they can do that offers the potential of changing the delivery of service in communication disorders.

Microcomputers are so called not only because they incorporate microprocessor technology but because they are small. The prefix "micro" differentiates them from minis and mainframes. In terms of memory capacity, however, they are as "big" as what we used to consider mainframes, and they keep getting "bigger." As integrated circuits are reduced in size, large computers are made more powerful and microcomputers perform all the functions of the previous generation of "large" machines. This trend will continue. Microcomputers will continue to become more powerful.

Like all computers, micros have a central processing unit (CPU) that is the "brains" of the machine. The CPU in currently available hardware is a group of logic circuits on a single chip. In addition to the CPU, memory is necessary in a computer for data storage and retrieval. Furthermore, all computers need programs (or software) to tell the CPU the sequence of operations, that is, what to do and when to do it. Programs for microcomputers are available on cassette tapes and floppy disks, which are coated with magnetic material. Disks have an advantage over magnetic tape as a storage media. Information stored on disks can be randomly accessed, whereas tape access is sequential, hence considerably slower. A means for getting information into and out of the machine must also be provided. The nature of these input/output (I/O) devices influences how a user can interact with a computer. Typically, data are entered through a keyboard, thus requiring at the very minimum that the user be able to recognize symbols of some kind. For most programs the user must be able to read. Using a keyboard, moreover, requires good motoric control in addition to being able to read.

RECENT INNOVATIONS IN MICROCOMPUTER TECHNOLOGY

How you interface with a machine can influence your perception of it. Negroponte (1979, p. 5) has pointed out:

> Such startling advances and cost reductions are occurring in microelectronics that we believe future systems will not be characterized by their memory size or processing speed. Instead, the human interface will become the major measure, calibrated in very subjective units, so sensory and personalized that it will be evaluated by feelings and perceptions. Is it easy to use? Does it feel good? Is it pleasurable?

A keyboard is no longer necessary for a user to interact with a computer. Input devices are now available that have changed the way we can interface with microcomputers. There are touch-sensitive screens, game paddles, joysticks, light pens, button panels, even eye movement sensors, and new devices are being developed. Although some of them are still expensive, they will not remain so. Reduced cost will make them available to the very young and the severely handicapped. Additionally, it is possible to develop microcomputer courseware (i.e., software for educational purposes) that can accept input from a broad range of devices. These devices can, in fact, be individually designed to suit the needs of the handicapped user.

Computer output has changed too. Text produced on a screen or by a printer is only one of the myriad ways a computer can output information. Color graphics is a good example of nontext output. In the case of the Apple II microcomputer, there is a peripheral input device for generating graphics, the Apple Graphics Tablet. This device and its related software allows the user to create and store images in six high resolution colors using a 53,760-dot display in a matrix 280 dots wide by 192 dots high. You "draw" right on the tablet with the attached pen and watch while images appear on the screen. With graphics instead of text, we can design programs for nonreaders.

If graphics were the only nontext output available, we would be restricted to various forms of matching tasks with nonreaders, but microcomputers can also talk. Two basic types of speech synthesizers are currently marketed for use with microcomputers. One uses phoneme generation, the other makes a digital recording of speech phrases. The Echo II® and the Votrax® are examples of phoneme synthesizers.

Some readers may be familiar with the quality of synthesized speech from having heard their children's Speak and Spell® toys or the HandiVoice®. Although these devices are memory efficient, they have a "computer accent." For applications where this "accent" is a problem, speech digitizers can provide more realistic sounds. The Mountain Computer SuperTalker is an example of a digitizing unit that interfaces with the Apple II. At its highest digitization rate, which produces the best quality, the SuperTalker samples a speaker's input at 4,096 bytes per second. The speech produced by the device retains the intonational patterns of the human speaker whose voice was digitized, stored, and reproduced. The price paid for better quality speech synthesis is two-fold: much more memory is required, and programming flexibility is severely restricted. For comparison, the Echo II uses 2 to 40 bytes of memory per spoken word, and the Mountain Computer SuperTalker uses 500 to 4,000 (Munro, 1982).

DEVELOPMENT OF AUDIBLE, MICROCOMPUTER ASSISTED INSTRUCTIONAL PROGRAMS

We first became intrigued with developing microcomputer based, audible, computer assisted instruction (CAI) in the fall of 1979. We wondered whether receptive language tests and programs, such as the Wilson Initial Syntax Program (Wilson, 1972) could be adapted to microcomputer administration. The WISP is a totally receptive language program that consists of 25 lessons covering basic phrase structure rules and single based transformations. The WISP has been used with mentally retarded and learning disabled children (Bannatyne, 1974; Fristoe, 1976) as well as other language disabled children and has been effective in remediating syntactic deficits.

Hardware

By late 1979 the Apple II microcomputer was fast becoming an educational favorite. Schools were purchasing TRS 80s in large numbers for their computer literacy courses, but Apples were more popular with educators looking for a broad range of courseware. This factor influenced our decision to purchase an Apple. The most important consideration was the graphics capabilities of the Apple, and the availability of graphics and speech generation peripherals. For program development we purchased the following equipment:

Apple II Plus 48K Microcomputer with two disk drives
Apple Graphics Tablet
Mountain Hardware (now Mountain Computer) SuperTalker

IDS 440 Paper Tiger Printer (with graphics capability)
Sony 13-inch color TV
Radiofrequency modulator unit
Amplifier/mixer and headphones

The Graphics Tablet, a $795 peripheral, and the printer are necessary for developing courseware but are not needed by a user to run it. Today, the configuration of equipment minus these peripherals costs about $3,000.

Software

Using the software supplied with the Apple Graphics Tablet is too slow for testing or training young children because the computer has to retrieve data stored on the disk (approximately 4.5 seconds) for each new graphic load (every second picture). Leslie Smith, then a senior in the Computer Science program at the University of Vermont, worked during the spring of 1980 on an assembly language utility program that would speed the process of stimulus presentation to provide storage of more pictures in active memory. The program, as developed, consisted of two parts. The first part was used in conjunction with the Apple Graphics Tablet. In the Apple computer each dot on the TV screen corresponds to a number (or address) in the Apple computer's memory. The program written by Smith isolated one small but critical portion of the TV screen (representing the "picture"); located the area in the computer that represented this picture, copied the numbers (representing the picture) into another area of the computer's memory (much smaller than the "screen" area of the computer's memory), and then compressed (codified number patterns) this information in an effort to reduce further the amount of memory needed to store this graphic information. The pattern of numbers is saved on the disk as a binary file. The second portion of the program involves the use of the system. The binary files representing, say, 25 pictures, are loaded into different areas of the Apple's memory. When one of these pictures is needed on the screen, the critical pattern of numbers is taken from the data storage area of the computer and transferred to the area of the computer that represents the screen. As soon as this has been done, the picture appears on the screen. Maximum time is less than one half second, and the number of searches to disk is reduced.

Courseware

The first courseware we developed was a prototype receptive syntax test. The program consisted of 10 sets of three lexically similar, grammatically contrasting pictures for testing comprehension of "in," "on," and "under." By using the assembly language graphics coding software in our test, only two loads were required during test administration. To maintain the child's interest during loads, an animated clown appeared, spoke the words "Good working," and remained on the screen while the computer was loading.

Because we wanted to test young children, we needed an input device other than a keyboard. In fact we did not want the children to be aware of the microcomputer. A touch-sensitive screen overlay would have been ideal for our purposes, because we could then have had the instructions say "Touch! The ball is in the box." However, our budget did not allow for the purchase of this device, so we designed a pushbutton panel to attach to the monitor and feed response data directly into the CPU. The panel was constructed of heavy gauge aluminum with three heavy duty, normally off, spring loaded switches. The button switches were located directly below the monitor screen in line with the area allocated for picture presentation. Figure 1 shows the equipment configuration used with this courseware. One of the 10 sets of stimulus pictures appears on the screen.

After our prototype receptive test was developed, our first question was whether this courseware could be successfully used with young children. We also wanted to know whether there would be a

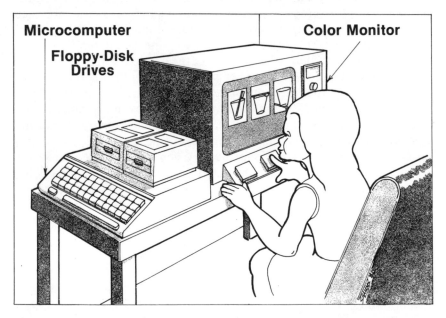

Figure 1.   Configuration of equipment used with the courseware.

difference in performance on a live version of the receptive test versus the computer assisted version. Finally, we wondered which method children prefer. To measure this, we asked children to choose either a live or computer administered test procedure after exposure to both methods.

Results

We used five normally developing children and 10 language impaired children in our sample (Fox, 1980; Fox and Wilson, 1981). All the children interacted positively with the computer. On the other hand, two refused all live testing. Only one child chose live over computer testing after exposure to both. There was no difference between the live and computer administered scores.

This study demonstrates the feasibility of using microcomputer administered software for testing the receptive use of prepositions and, by inference, other language measures. Using vocabulary, syntax, and concept testing courseware in screening programs offers a viable and less expensive alternative to live testing. Similarly, audible tests could be developed to test aphasic adults. Obviously, if we consider the design of tests that use text instead of or in addition to graphics, we can develop microcomputer tests that measure receptive and expressive skills. For example, a program could present the sentence "He is a boy" with the instruction to make the same words into a question. The program could accept the child's response, analyze it, score it, and provide a test report.

Computer testing, in addition to its economic appeal, offers the advantage of always presenting stimuli in the same manner. Consistent presentation of stimuli eliminates the possibility of having test results influenced by the examiner's behavior. This factor can be especially critical in bilingual language assessment (Wilson and Fox, 1981a, 1982). During computer assisted testing, data are collected and subsequently analyzed and reported accurately. This arrangement is not always possible with live testing. Programs can also be developed that prescribe treatment after testing. Indeed microcomputer courseware for training will probably include pretraining and posttraining tests. Assessment after all is simply one step in the process of teaching.

DEVELOPMENT OF COMPREHENSION
TRAINING PROGRAM FOR PREPOSITIONS

After we had established that microcomputer courseware could be used in comprehension testing, we turned our attention to developing comprehension training programs. Comprehension is critical to the development of communication systems, as Winitz (1981) has pointed out. Studies have demonstrated that comprehension training can improve expressive as well as receptive performance (Cuvo and Riva, 1980; Ruder, Hermann, and Schiefelbusch, 1977; Wilson, 1977; Winitz and Reeds, 1975). Other studies have demonstrated that modeling procedures wherein the child hears a construction in an appropriate context seem to be more effective than imitation procedures in language development (Courtright and Courtright, 1976, 1979; Harris and Hassemer, 1972; Zimmerman and Pike, 1972; Zimmerman and Rosenthal, 1974).

Understanding what is heard is fundamental to communication. Children acquire language by using their innate language capacities and listening skills. We believed that microcomputer courseware could be developed to assist the speech-language pathologist and the classroom teacher in providing the necessary systematic exposure and structured linguistic environment to help children to acquire the rules of language.

Courseware

As we began designing language training courseware, we wondered what antecedent and consequent events should be included to ensure program success. Therefore we designed training courseware for the same prepositions we had used in our test: "in," "on," and "under." We decided first to investigate what feedback procedures would be effective. To measure these effects we designed a single subject, multibaseline study (Wilson and Fox, 1981b). Single subject, multibaseline designs can be used to analyze specific components of an instruction design in an efficient manner (Cuvo, 1979; Strain and Shores, 1979). The courseware we developed did not use any antecedent instructional components. The two feedback techniques we compared were the only instructional components in the courseware, which was designed to teach the prepositions "in" and "on."

The two feedback approaches used in the comprehension training courseware were knowledge of the correct response (KCR) and cueing of the correct response (CCR). In KCR the learner is always told the correct answer, through reinforcement when correct or through information feedback when incorrect. In CCR a correct answer is reinforced, but when an error has been made the learner is given a cue to the correct response and then gets a second chance to respond.

Program Testing and Results

The subject was a 38-month old language delayed girl. Before training, we used a 45-item (15 sets of in/on/under pictures) preposition test to assess comprehension of "in," "on," and "under." We terminated baseline testing on the second day because the child's scores were similar on both days. Ten of the picture stimulus sets were used in training, and five were held as controls.

There were three training segments, each of which was followed by readministration of the 45-item test. "In" was trained first. The 45-item test given after training revealed that the child had learned "in" but did not comprehend "on" and "under." Similarly, after "on" training test scores revealed that she was comprehending both "in" and "on" but not "under." A final training sequence mixed "in" and "on." On the final test she demonstrated mastery of "in" (10/10 = 100%) and "on" (8/10 = 80%) on the trained items. Furthermore, on the final test she correctly responded to all the "in" stimulus items from the five untrained sets and correctly identified three of the untrained "on" stimuli. The two untrained items she identified incorrectly had never been identified correctly in any of the five test sessions. Since at no time did she correctly "guess" either of the items, the graphics for these two might have been ambiguous to her. Her "in" and "on" scores in the posttest are in contrast to those for "under," which were 2/10 for the sets used in the training sessions and 2/5 for the graphics presented as controls.

This study showed that audible and visual feedback is an effective teaching technique. Similar results have been obtained with nonaudible print feedback and KCR (Anderson, Kulhavy, and Andre, 1971; Gilman, 1969; Tait, Hartley, and Anderson, 1973). Since there was no difference in the effectiveness of the two feedback methods, both can be incorporated in future curricular programs for receptive language instruction. Total programs should, of course, use a variety of antecedent and consequent events that have been found to be effective in studies such as the one described.

OTHER APPLICATIONS

Vocabulary Building and Concept Training

Vocabulary building and concept training can also be accomplished with microcomputer courseware. For example, we have recently developed a 50-word vocabulary program that uses a variety of cueing and feedback techniques performed by an animated green "Blob" who has feet to jump and run. He can also tuck in his legs and roll around. Sometimes when he jumps too high, he squishes up when he lands and makes a funny face. He opens and closes his mouth when he makes sounds and talks. Counters built into the program keep track of the child's score.

The program itself has six levels of training and is intended for use with young mildly handicapped children or older severely or profoundly mentally retarded children. This program as well as the others we are developing would also be appropriate for use in an English as a second language curriculum. This program is currently being field tested.

Treatment of Autistic Children

Microcomputer courseware may in the future offer new hope for the autistic child. Treatment for autistic children has generally not been successful and the prognosis for them is guarded (Magrab, 1976). Many authorities now agree that language deficits are central to the autistic child's disturbed social interactions. Investigators have suggested that the social and behavioral abnormalities observed in autistic children arise as secondary consequences to a primary deficit of language (Bartak, Rutter, and Cox, 1975; Rutter, 1968; Rutter and Bartak, 1971). Wing and Gould (1979) recently found that children regarded as "aloof" could be characterized by poor language comprehension. Colby (1973, p. 258) has stated: "There are students of autism who consider non-speaking autistic children to be fundamentally withdrawn from people and hence not acquiring language. We feel it is the other way around: they have so much difficulty with language they withdraw . . . ."

Thus, in the autistic child, disturbances in pragmatics—that is, social and communicative interactive behavior—appear to rest on noncomprehension of the structural aspects of communication. If social development in the autistic child is language based, an effective language intervention program is needed to improve social interaction. Microcomputer courseware promises to fulfill this need. Given the autistic child's difficulties with human interaction, the task of rule induction would seem to be complicated by the presence of another person, who expects communication to take place. To date syntax comprehension training either has not been done with these children, as is the case with the operant approach that uses imitation as the basis for communication, or has been done by human trainers.

By using microcomputer administered courseware for syntactic training, the task is solely centered on rule induction. A number of authors have even cited the autistic child's fascination with machines and willingness to work with them (Colby, 1973; Doherty and Swisher, 1978; Howe, 1979). Quality microcomputer courseware can capitalize on this fascination in a learning context. Microcomputer courseware may well meet the needs of improving autistic children's language comprehension in a way that human instruction cannot.

Uses in Special Education

Certainly one use for microcomputer courseware in our field is in language comprehension testing and training. These programs offer special promise not only for autistic children, but also for mentally retarded and learning disabled youngsters with interactive language disorders that require intensive intervention. Microcomputer courseware can provide the tutorial instruction necessary for these children to acquire lexical items, concepts, and grammatical rules. Programs could also be developed to teach comprehension of pragmatic behaviors. The use of microcomputer courseware to provide tutorial instruction that human teachers frequently find boring, albeit necessary, frees teachers to provide social communication activities that require human interaction. With microcomputer courseware available, for example, in the area of language comprehension, the speech-language pathologist can concentrate on the development of pragmatic abilities. Not only can microcomputers be used in language comprehension testing and training, they can be used to administer reading and math programs designed for learning disabled youngsters. Hannaford and Sloane (1981, p. 54) have stated this position as follows: "For special educators, the microcomputer can act as a tireless teacher's aide, allowing highly interactive learning to take place at the individual student's rate of learning."

Other Applications: Aphasia and Motorically Handicapped Individuals

In addition to the treatment of autistic children and uses in special education, there are other applications of microcomputers. Aphasia treatment is one example (Mills and Langmore, 1980). In other areas, the employment of microcomputers as prosthetic devices seems to be limited more by the imaginations of users than by inherent characteristics of the machine. For example, new developments in microcomputer technology now offer the promise of designing effective and efficient communication systems for the motorically handicapped. Because microcomputers can be interfaced with speech synthesizers, speech-language pathologists have equipment available on which to experiment with various communication programs.

For the reader interested in learning more about the range of microcomputer applications to aid handicapped persons, the IEEE's Proceedings of the Johns Hopkins First National Search for Applications of Personal Computing to Aid the Handicapped (Hazan, 1981) provides an excellent overview. Ninety-seven of the prize winning entries are described in this volume. The applications vary from prosthetic devices such as augmentative communication and environmental controls to training software.

FUTURE PROSPECTS

Over the next decade as microcomputer use in education increases, the need for quality courseware will become acute. Speech-language pathologists need to be aware of the various clinical roles microcomputer courseware can fill. If the microcomputer is, as many believe, going to revolutionize the teaching/learning process (Evans, 1980; Papert, 1980), then special educators must make certain that communicatively handicapped children are INCLUDED not EXCLUDED. This can only happen if speech-language pathologists have knowledge of microcomputer applications with handicapped children and those who are directly responsible for the implementation of individualized education programs (IEPs) have skills in microcomputer use. Similarly, in the area of aphasia rehabilitation, microcomputer courseware can intensify the level of training. For rural homebound aphasics, microcomputer courseware may well be the only possible daily intervention.

Over the past 2 years as we have presented workshops and papers across the country, we have noted a growing acceptance of microcomputers as clinical tools. When we first began our development work some of our colleagues did not believe microcomputers would be used by clinicians in our field. Computers were regarded solely as administrative and research tools. That certainly has changed! Few now doubt that microcomputer courseware can assist us in our clinical work.

If speech-language pathologists do not realize the potential of microcomputer applications in our field, someone else will, and we will find ourselves as we have before, bemoaning the "invasion of our territory." As we move toward the twenty-first century, we must make strides toward learning about and incorporating new technology into our programs for handicapped persons. This chapter has only glossed over important clinical applications of microcomputer technology. Professionals in the field must accept the challenge new technologies pose if we are to meet best the needs of the communicatively impaired people we serve.

REFERENCES

Anderson, R., Kulhavy, R., and Andre, T. 1971. Feedback procedures in programmed instruction. J. Educ. Psychol. 62:148–156.
Bannatyne, A. 1974. Programs, materials and techniques. J. Learn. Disabilities 7:6–7.

Bartak, L., Rutter, N., and Cox, A. 1975. A comparative study of infantile autism and specific developmental receptive language disorder. I. The children. Br. J. Psychiatr. 126:127–145.

Colby, K. 1973. The rationale for computer-based treatment of language difficulties in nonspeaking autistic children. J. Autism Child. Schizophrenia 3:245–260.

Courtright, J., and Courtright, I. 1976. Imitative modeling as a theoretical base for instructing language-disordered children. J. Speech Hear. Res. 19:665–663.

Courtright, J., and Courtright, I. 1979. Imitative modeling as a language intervention strategy: The effects of two mediating variables. J. Speech Hear. Res. 22:389–402.

Cuvo, A. 1979. Multiple-baseline design in instructional research: Pitfalls of measurement and procedural advantages. Am. J. Ment. Defic. 84:219–228.

Cuvo, A., and Riva, N. 1980. Generalization and transfer between comprehension and production: A comparison of retarded and nonretarded persons. J. Appl. Behav. Anal. 13:315–331.

Doherty, L., and Swisher, L. 1978. Children with autistic behaviors. In: F. Minifie and L. L. Lloyd (eds.), Communicative and Cognitive Abilities—Early Behavioral Assessment. University Park Press, Baltimore.

Evans, C. 1980. The Micro Millennium. Viking Press, New York.

Fox, B. 1980. A study comparing live and computer administered receptive syntax items testing the prepositions in, on, and under. Unpublished master's thesis. University of Vermont, Burlington.

Fox, B., and Wilson, M. 1981. Microcomputer administered receptive language testing: A new alternative. Unpublished manuscript, 1981.

Fristoe, M. 1976. Language intervention systems: Programs published in kit form. In: L. L. Lloyd (ed.), Communication Assessment and Intervention Strategies, pp. 813–859. University Park Press, Baltimore.

Gilman, A. 1969. Comparison of several feedback methods for correcting errors by computer-assisted instruction. J. Educ. Psychol. 60:503–508.

Hannaford, A., and Sloane, E. 1981. Microcomputers: Powerful learning tools with proper programming. Teach. Except. Child. 14:54–57.

Harris, M., and Hassemer, W. 1972. Some factors affecting the complexity of children's sentences: The effects of modeling, age, sex and bilingualism. J. Exp. Child Psychol. 13:447–455.

Hazan, P. (ed.). 1981. Proceedings of the Johns Hopkins First National Search for Applications of Personal Computing to Aid the Handicapped, IEEE Computer Society. Computer Society Press, New York.

Howe, J. 1979. Using computers to teach children with communication difficulties: A new deal? DAI Research Paper no. 111. Department of Artificial Intelligence, University of Edinburgh, Edinburgh, UK.

Magrab, P. 1976. Psychosocial function: Normal development—infantile autism. In: R. Johnston and P. Magrab (eds.), Developmental Disorders: Assessment, Treatment, Education. University Park Press, Baltimore.

Mills, R., and Langmore, S. 1980. A microcomputer system in aphasia rehabilitation. Scientific exhibit presented to the Annual Convention of the American Speech-Language-Hearing Association, Detroit.

Munro, A. 1982. An overview of speech synthesizers. Softalk, May.

Negroponte, N. 1979. Prologue. In: R. Bolt (ed.), Spatial Data Management. MIT Press, Cambridge, Mass.

Papert, S. 1980. Mindstorms. Basic Books, New York.

Ruder, K., Hermann, P., and Schiefelbusch, R. 1977. Effects of verbal imitation and comprehension training on verbal production. J. Psycholinguist. Res. 6:59–72.

Rutter, M. 1968. Concepts of autism: A review of research. J. Child Psychol. Psychiatr. 9:1–25.

Rutter, M., and Bartak, L. 1971. Causes of infantile autism: Some considerations from recent research. J. Autism Child. Schizophrenia 1:20–32.

Strain, P., and Shores, R. 1979. Additional comments on multiple-baseline designs in instructional research. Am. J. Ment. Defic. 84:229–234.

Tait, K., Hartley, J., and Anderson, R. 1973. Feedback procedures in computer-assisted arithmetic instruction. Br. J. Educ. Psychol. 43:161–171.

Wilson, M. 1972. Wilson Initial Syntax Program. Educators Publishing Service, Cambridge, Mass.

Wilson, M. 1977. Syntax Remediation, A Generative Grammar Approach to Language Development. Educators Publishing Service, Cambridge, Mass.

Wilson, M., and Fox, B. 1981a. The bilingual computer! Promise of the eighties. Guest Editorial, Asha 23:651–652.

Wilson, M., and Fox, B. 1981b. A study of feedback effects in microcomputer administered receptive language training. Unpublished manuscript.

Wilson, M., and Fox, B. 1982. Computer administered bilingual language assessment and intervention. Except. Child. 49:145–149.

Wing, L., and Gould, J. 1979. Severe impairments of social interaction and associated abnormalities in children: Epidemiology and classification. J. Autism Dev. Disord. 9:11–29.

Winitz, H. 1981. Nonlinear learning and language teaching. In: H. Winitz (ed.), The Comprehension Approach to Foreign Language Instruction. Newbury House, Rowley, Mass.

Winitz, H., and Reeds, J. 1975. Comprehension and Problem Solving as Strategies for Language Training. Mouton, The Hague.

Zimmerman, B., and Pike, E. 1972. Effects of modeling and reinforcement on the acquisition and generalization of question-asking behavior. Child Dev. 43:892–907.

Zimmerman, B., and Rosenthal, T. 1974. Observational learning of rule-governed behavior by children. Psychol. Bull. 81:29–42.

Index

Academic success, stimulus-
response for, 2–7
Accountability, 23
government assistance fostering,
12–14
Achievement, *see* Language
achievement
Acknowledgment, 83, 84, 85
Activities
communicative atmosphere
created by, 88–93
generalization, 18
goal directed, 37–38
learning through, 44–45
Adjectives, 32–33
Affective agnosia, 188
Affective-prosodic deblocker, 191,
193, 195–196, 198, 199, 201
Affirmation, in lexical items for
augmentative communication,
227
Agglutination, principle of, 222
American sign language (ASL), 212
Amerind, 222
Anosognosia for speech, in fluent
aphasics, 170
Aphasia
apraxia of speech with, 165
aprosodias, 188, 189
Boston school of, 166
Broca's, 188, 189, 192, 193
deblocking for, 193, 195–196,
197
classification of, 166–167
deblocking, 165, 183–184
affective-prosodic, 191, 193,
195–196, 198, 199, 201
rudimentary linguistic, 191, 193,
195–196, 198, 199, 200,
201–202
visual-spatial-holistic, 191, 193,
195–196, 198, 199, 200, 201,
202
see also minor hemisphere
mediation, *below*

fluent, 166, 167
assessment in, 176–177
communication style of,
167–176
compensatory efforts in,
170–171
comprehension in, 168–169
content awareness in, 170
monitor as communication style
of, 173–174
rambler as communication style
of, 171–173
self-monitoring in, 169–170
significant others involved with,
177
unknowing compensator as
communication style of,
174–176
microcomputers for, 245, 246
minor hemisphere mediation for,
184
for Broca's aphasia, 193,
195–196, 197
dominant hemisphere
participation in speech,
184–185, 188, 189
for facilitation of expressive
language, 192–193, 197,
201–202
for facilitation of receptive
language, 190–192, 194–196,
198–200
goals of, 188
minor hemisphere participation
in speech, 184–188, 189
for Wernicke's aphasia,
197–202
nonfluent, 165, 166
treatment, 164–166, 183–184
communicative interplay,
155–157
intensive stimulation approach,
146–147
intersystemic reorganization,
183, 184

Aphasia—*continued*
  intrasystemic reorganization,
    183, 184
  unconscious generation of
    spontaneous language and,
    146, 153
  see also deblocking and minor
    hemispheric mediation, *above*
  Wernicke's, 166, 189, 190,
    192–193
  deblocking for, 197–202
Apple II microcomputer, 237,
    238–241
Application activity, generalization
    obtained by, 18
Apraxia of speech, 165
Aprosodias, 188, 189
Articles, development of, 3–4
Assessment
  of achievement, 30, 31–35
  of comprehension, 46–53
  continuous recordings for, 73–74
  elicited imitation for, 47
  in emotionally handicapped
    children, 130–131
  of improvements, 73–76
  of language production, 39–40
  language sampling for, 75, 76
  of perceptual skills, 130
  of production, 49–51
  of semantic development, 86
  of social skills, 130
  structural observation for, 75, 76
  of syntax, 46–47, 86
  two-word stage and, 83, 85–86, 87
  see also Interactive model; Tests
    and testing
Atmosphere of delight, *see*
    Spontaneous language
Attention, as instructional strategy,
    68–69
Augmentative communication
  decision making process in,
    206–207, 208
  functionally based nesting model
    for, 212–213
  lexical items for, 207, 209, 210,
    211–214
    affirmation and negation in, 227
    back-channel responses for, 230
    body parts in, 228
    colors in, 227–228

constraints of symbol system in
      selection of, 217–221, 222
    discourse principles and,
      229–231
    evaluation of, 221–229
    frequency of use of, 224
    here and now reflected by,
      222–223
    iconicity of, 217–218
    idiosyncratic signal system
      expressing, 223–224
    information conveyed by,
      224–225
    intelligibility of, 221
    interest value of, 213, 228–229
    for multiword combinations,
      222
    nonlinguistic support for,
      225–226
    nonverbal communication and,
      223–224
    opposites in, 226–227
    peer interaction fostered by,
      226
    perceptual complexity of, 219
    reinforcement value of, 225
    social organization devices for,
      230
    topographical similarity of,
      219–220
    variety of communicative
      functions coded by, 221–222
    word pool for, 214–217
  potential population for, 210, 211
Autistic child, 125–126
  cognitive development in, 131
  expansion for, 138
  feedback technique for, 139–140
  microcomputers for, 244
  perceptual deficiency in, 130
  teaching language to, 123, 128
Auxiliaries, 34
  contractible, 3–4
  data based language programs
    and, 15
  uncontractible, 3, 6–7

Back-channel responses, for lexicon
    for augmentative
    communication, 230
Backward chaining, 16
Blissymbolics, 218–219, 222, 226

Bloom-Lahey model, for
emotionally handicapped
children with language
disorders, 125–129
Body parts, in lexical items for
augmentative communication,
228
Boston Diagnostic Aphasia Exam,
176
Boston School of Aphasia, 166
Broca's aphasia, 188, 189, 192, 193
deblocking, 193, 195–196, 197
Broca's aprosodia, 188, 189

CADL, see Communication Abilities
in Daily Living
Calling/greeting, 82, 84, 85
Catenatives, 112, 114–115
Causative verbs, 32–33
Central processing unit (CPU), 236
Chunking, remembering facilitated
by, 52
Classroom
comprehension and production in,
50
language testing in, 49
Clause juxtaposition, routine events
facilitating the use of,
110–111
Clinic, language testing in, 49
Clinician-as-communicator, 103–104
Cognition, in the developmental
process, 61
Colors, in lexical items for
augmentative communication,
227–228
Communication, teaching language
through, 36–38
Communicative Abilities in Daily
Living (CADL), 177
Communication styles, of fluent
aphasics, 167–176
Communicative context
linguistic context, 99–100,
113–118
for conveying communicative
intent, 102–103
materials for, 109
nonlinguistic context, 100
clinician-as-communicator and,
103–104
linguistic context and, 102–103

listener knowledge and,
101–103
listener needs adaptation and,
101–103
perceptual support and,
100–101, 105–108
strategies of preparatory to
speech acts, 109–112
nonlinguistic support, 105–108
Communicative intent, 82, 84
Communicative interplay,
spontaneous language and,
155–157
Compensatory efforts, in fluent
aphasics, 170–171
Competing auditory message,
comprehension and
production and, 50, 52
Complex concepts, 48, 51
Complex sentences, routine events
facilitating the use of, 110–111
Comprehension, 168
assessment of, 46–53
in fluent aphasics, 169
microcomputers and
testing, 238–241, 245
training, 241–243, 245
strategy for teaching, 71
training, 40–41
Computer assisted instruction
(CAI), 238–241
Computer output, 237
Computers, see Microcomputers
Concepts
comprehension and production of,
48–50
microcomputers for, 243–244
teaching, 51–52
Conclusions, workbooks for, 52
Content, 67–68, 80
in Bloom-Lahey model, 125–126
in emotionally handicapped child,
132, 133–134
disorders, 126–127
in fluent aphasics, 170
Context
meaning varying according to, 62
spontaneous speech and, 158–159
workbooks for, 52
see also Interactive model
Contingent directives, language
facilitation by, 108

Continuous recording, language improvement evaluated by, 73–74
Contractible auxiliary, development of, 3–4
Contractible copula, development of, 3–4
Copula, 3–4
Criterion referenced tests, 64–67
Cueing, aphasia treated with, 164–165
Cueing of the correct response (CCR), as feedback approach, 242–243
Curriculum, *see* Emotionally handicapped child; Language curriculum

Data based language programs, *see* Language programs
Deblocking, *see* Aphasia
Delight, atmosphere of, *see* Spontaneous language
Detailing, 84, 85
Developmental approach, 3–5, 25
  achievement interpreted in, 30, 31–35
  communicative approach, 36–38
  errors in language development revealing flaws in, 29–30
  to expressive language, 39–41
  horizontal, 4–5
  instruction based on, 61–63
  language input procedures prescribed by, 30–31
  premises of, 26–28, 33, 34, 35
  in selection of lexical items for augmentative communication, 209, 211–214
  vertical, 3–4
  see also Language curriculum
Developmental index, language improvement evaluation and, 75–76
Diagnosis, criterion referenced testing and, 65
Dialectical model, of development, 62
Directions, 84, 85
  learning to give, 111
  workbooks for, 52

Directives
  initiating, 111–112
  as language facilitation stretegy, 7, 108, 110–111, 113
Direct techniques, for emotionally handicapped children, 138–139
Discourse principle, 7, 8
  in the selection and organization of a nonspeaker's lexicon, 229–231
Discrimination, as learning strategy, 70
Dominant (left) hemisphere, speech and, 184–185, 188, 189
Dual meanings, jokes used for, 52

Echolalia, in emotionally handicapped children, 128
Echo II, 237–238
Education for All Handicapped Children Act (PL 94-142), 12–13
  see also Individualized education program
Elective mutism, in emotionally handicapped children, 129
Elicited imitation
  as language facilitation strategy, 113, 114–115
  language production assessed with, 47
Eliciting language, facilitating language in emotionally handicapped child with, 138–139
Ellipsis discourse rule, *see* Discourse principle
Emotionally handicapped child, 123
  assessing language production in, 129–130
  Bloom-Lahey model for, 125–129
  content disorders in, 126–127
  curriculum for, 133–134
    eliciting in, 138–139
    expansion in, 137–138, 139
    feedback in, 139–141
    mapping in, 135–136
    modeling in, 136–137, 139
    working alliance established in, 134–135

form disorders in, 127–128
goals in teaching, 133
interpretive work with, 132–133
use disorders in, 128–129
working alliance establishment
    and, 123–125
Environmental demands, language
    performance and, 154–155
Errorless learning, 15–16
Errors
    data based language programs
        and, 21–22
    in language acquisition, 29–30
    learning without, 15–16
    in testing comprehension, 47
Evaluation procedures, see
    Assessment; Tests and testing
Event representations, 105–106
Expansion
    for emotionally handicapped
        child, 137–138, 139
    language facilitation by, 110–111,
        113
Expatiation, 116
Expressive language
    development of, 39–41
    minor hemispheric mediation
        facilitating, 192–193, 197,
        201–202
    training, 34
Extension activity, generalization
    obtained by, 18
Eye contact, 68
    techniques for facilitating, 15

Familiar routines, language use
    facilitated by, 106–108
Feedback
    facilitating language in
        emotionally handicapped
        child with, 139–141
    in the presentation of language
        material by computer,
        242–243
Feelings, expressing, 84, 85
Fluent aphasia, see Aphasia
Forced production, 35–36, 38
Foreign language, see Second
    language
Form, 80
    in Bloom-Lahey model, 125–126

in emotionally handicapped child,
    127–128, 132, 134
Formal testing procedure, 73, 76
Form disorders, in emotionally
    handicapped, 127–128, 132,
    134
Free play, generalization training
    and, 19
Function, in language acquisition,
    67–68
Functionally based nesting model,
    for augmentative
    communication, 212–213

Generalization, 18
    data based language programs
        and, 17–19
Gestural imitation, 82, 84
Goal directed activity,
    communicative centered
    activities including, 37–38
Grammatical morpheme, 34
    data based language programs
        and, 18–19
    development of, 3–4
Group training sessions, for
    emotionally handicapped
    children, 139

Handicapped, microcomputers for,
    245, 246
    see also Emotionally handicapped
        child
Handi Voice, 238
Hemisphere mediation, see Aphasia
Horizontal developmental approach,
    to language training, 4–5

Iconicity, of symbol sets, 217–218
Ideographic processing, minor
    hemisphere and, 185–186, 187
Imaging, in aphasia treatment, 186
Imitation
    elicited, 47, 113, 114–115
    gestural, 82, 84
    as learning strategy, 69–70
    as measure of language
        production, 46–47
    vocal, 82, 84
Incident description, 84, 85
Incorrect responses, see Errors

Indirect teaching, for emotionally
    handicapped children,
    138–139
Individual education program (IEP),
    12–13, 23
  data based language program
    achieving, see Language
    programs
  goals of and language learning
    processes, 71–73
  language curriculum and, 61, 62,
    63
  microcomputers and, 246
Infinitives, 111
Informal testing procedure, 73
Information processing, of listener,
    102
Input devices, for microcomputers,
    237
Intensive stimulation approach, to
    aphasia, 146–147
Interactive model, 80–81
  assessment in, 81–86
    language sampling for, 82–86
    standard procedures for, 82
    in two-word stage, 83, 85–86,
      87
  treatment in, 86, 88
    for one-word level of
      communicating, 88–90
    for prelinguistic child, 88–90
    for two- and three-word
      combinations, 92–93
    for two-word level of
      communicating, 90–91
Internal states, describing, 111
Interpersonal monitoring, in fluent
    aphasics, 169
Intersystemic reorganization, for
    aphasia, 183, 184
Intransitive verbs, 32–33
Intrapersonal monitoring, in fluent
    aphasics, 169
Intrasystemic reorganization, for
    aphasia, 183, 184
Irregular past tense, 3–4
Irregular third person singular, 3–4

Jokes, for dual meaning
    understanding, 52
Juxtaposing clauses, routine events
    facilitating, 110–111

Klang associations, in emotionally
    handicapped children, 127
Knowledge, of listener, 101–103
Knowledge of the correct response
    (KCR), as feedback
    approach, 242–243

Labeling, 82, 83, 84
Language, language facilitation by,
    113–118
Language achievement, 27
  developmental approach and, 27,
    30, 31–35
Language acquisition, 28–30
  achievement and, 35
  in Bloom-Lahey model, 125–126
  curriculum for, see Language
    curriculum
  errors in, 29–30
  function and content in, 67–68
  language role in, 113–118
  minor hemisphere participation in,
    187
  social context of, 80–81, see also
    Interactive model
Language age, establishing for
    developmental model, 26–27
Language curriculum
  definition, 59–60
  evaluation procedures for, 73–76
  instruction strategies specified for,
    67–71
  language acquisition model
    specified in, 61–63
  outcomes of instruction specified
    for, 71–73
  target population specified for,
    63–67
  see also Emotionally handicapped
    child
Language input, developmental
    approach and, 30–31
Language intervention, 51–53,
    106–108
Language production
  evaluation of, 46–53
  exercises, 39–40
Language programs
  data based, 13
    accountability of, 13–14
    effectiveness of, 16–22
    evaluation of, 22–23

generalization in, 17–19
incorrect response and, 21–22
popularity of, 13–16
predetermined response in,
    19–20
scoring procedure, 16–17
task analysis, 15–16
packaged, 5–7
see also Microcomputers
Language sampling
as language assessment
    procedure, 75, 76
pragmatic behaviors elicited by,
    82–86
Language test, see Tests and testing
Language training, communicative
    approach to, 36–38
see also Naturalness, language
    training achieving
Laughter, language spontaneity and,
    154, 161
Learning strategies, see Strategies
    of learning
Levels, of language, 61–62
Levels of processing model, 45–46
Lexical items, see Augmentative
    communication
Linear learning, 32
Linguistic contexts, see
    Communicative context
Linguistic functions, of the
    dominant hemisphere, 185
Listener, adapting to needs of,
    101–103
Listener knowledge, 101–103
Locative action, coordination of,
    117–118
Logorrhea, fluent aphasic with, 171

Main idea, workbooks for, 52
Mapping, facilitating language in
    emotionally handicapped
    child with, 135–136
Matching, as learning strategy, 69
Melodic intonation therapy (MIT),
    aphasia treated with, 165, 184
Microcomputers, 236–237, 246
for aphasia, 245, 246
Apple II, 237, 238–241
for autistic children, 244
central processing unit of, 236

comprehension testing program
    with, 238–241, 245
comprehension training program
    with, 241–243, 245
computer assisted instruction
    with, 238–241
concept training from, 243–244
for handicapped, 245, 246
input devices for, 237
output, 237–238
for special education, 245
speech synthesizers of, 237–238
vocabulary building from, 243–244
Minor hemisphere mediation, see
    Aphasia
Modeling
for emotionally handicapped
    child, 136–137, 139
in interactive model, 86, 91
language facilitation by, 107, 113
Monitor, fluent aphasic as, 173–174
Morpheme, see Grammatical
    morpheme
Mothers, replicating input style of,
    99
see also Communicative context;
    Parents
Motor aphasia, see Broca's aphasia
Motor aprosodia, see Broca's
    aprosodia
Mountain Computer SuperTalker,
    238
Multimodality language retraining,
    in aphasic persons, 184

Naturalness, language training
    achieving, 6–7
parent-child interactions for, 7
play therapy for, 7–8
see also Stimulus-response
    intervention technique
Negation
coding, 112
in lexical items for augmentative
    communication, 227
Nondirective approach in training,
    7–8
Nonfluent aphasia, 165, 166
Nonlinguistic context, see
    Communicative context
Nonlinguistic support, 105–108
in selecting initial lexical items for

Nonlinguistic support—*continued*
augmentative communication,
225–226
Nonspeakers, language for, *see*
Augmentative communication
Nonverbal cues, in augmentative
communication, 223–224
Norm referenced tests, 64
Novel pictographs
aphasia treated by, 184
minor hemisphere activity
enhanced by, 186–187

Object permanence, 69, 82, 84
Objects
hiding, 112
violation of function and
manipulation of, 111–112
withholding, 111
One-word level of communicating,
treatment program on, 88–90
Open ended stimulus question, 7
Opposites, in lexical items for
augmentative communication,
226–227

PACE, *see* Promoting Aphasics'
Communicative Effectiveness
Packaged programs, for language
training, 5–7
Paraphrasing, teaching, 51
Parents
communicate skills of child from,
82
involvement of in interactive
model, 89
parent-child interaction studies,
7–8
replicating input style of, 99, *see
also* Communicative context
Peer interaction, lexical items in
augmentative communication
fostering, 226
Perceptual skills, assessing in
emotionally handicapped
children, 130
Perceptual support, 100–101,
105–108
for an utterance, 100–101
Performance contracting,
accountability and, 12–14

Phoneme synthesizers, of
microcomputers, 237–238
PICA, *see* Porch Index of
Communicative Ability
Picture pointing tasks,
comprehension tested with,
47
Pictorial stimuli, in aphasia
treatment, 186–187
Play
free, 19
in interactive model, 90–91
language instruction in context of,
62, 81
lexical items in augmentative
communication fostering, 226
structured, 8
symbolic, 82, 84
therapy, 7–8
Play therapy, 7–8
Plurals, development of, 3–4
Porch Index of Communicative
Ability (PICA), 176
Possessives, development of, 3–4
Pragmatics, 36–37, 66, 67, 80–81
measures of, 81–86
see also Interactive model
Prelinguistic communication, 88–90
see also Interactive model
Preprogrammed responses, data
based language program and,
19–20
Presentation, rate of for emotionally
handicapped, 140–141
Processing, levels of, 45–46
Production, *see* Language
production
Programs, *see* Language programs
Progressive endings
data based language programs
and, 18–19, 21
development of, 3–4, 34
Promoting Aphasics'
Communicative Effectiveness
(PACE), 197, 201
for unknowing compensators, 176
Prosodic features, in emotionally
handicapped children, 127
Protesting, 82, 83, 84, 85, 111–112
Public Law 94-142, *see* Education of
All Handicapped Children
Act

Pumping
   in language training, 154–155,
      156–157
   spontaneous language and, 161

Questions
   language facilitation by, 108, 113
   open ended stimulus, 7
   wh-, 112, 114–115

Rambler, fluent aphasic as, 171–173
Readiness test, 48
Receptive Expressive Emergent
      Language Scale (REEL), 82
Receptive language
   minor hemisphere mediation
      facilitating, 190–192, 194–196,
      197–200
   scale for, 82
Recognition
   comprehension tested with, 47
   teaching strategies organized
      under, 70–71
REEL, see Receptive Expressive
      Emergent Language Scale
Regular past tense, development of,
      3–4
Regular third person singular,
      development of, 3–4
Rehearsing, remembering facilitated
      by, 52
Reinforcement, see Stimulus-
      response intervention
      technique
Remembering, strategies to
      facilitate, 52
Repetition, 83, 84, 85
   for emotionally handicapped
      children, 137
Reporting, 83, 84, 85
Requesting, 82, 83, 84
   action, 84, 85
   information, 82–83, 84, 85
   objects, 84, 85
Responding, 83, 84, 85
   incorrect, 21–22
   preprogramming of correct, 19–20
Right (minor) hemisphere, see
      Aphasia
Role playing
   for fluent aphasia, 177
   for social awareness, 52

Routine
   familiar, 106–108
   violation of, 109–111
   word pool for augmentative
      communication and, 215
Rudimentary linguistic deblocker,
      191, 193, 195–196, 198, 199,
      200, 201–202

Salient stimulus, attention and,
      68–69
Second-language
   communicative activities for
      teaching, 38
   learning, 28–29
   unconscious generation of
      language and, 147
Self-criticism, in fluent aphasics, 170
Self-maintaining, 84, 85
Self-monitoring, in fluent aphasics,
      169
Semantics
   depth and breadth of, 62
   development of, 89–91, 86
   for language intervention, 51
   measures of comprehension of,
      46–47
Sensory modalities, selection of the
      appropriate, 140
Sequenced Inventory of
      Communication Development
      (SICD), 82
Shared knowledge, listener
      knowledge and, 101–102
Shared social scripts, 105
SICD, see Sequenced Inventory of
      Communication Development
Significant others, fluent aphasics
      and, 177
Social context
   of language, 61, 80–81
   of language instruction, 62
   see also Interactive model; Play
Social organization devices, for
      lexicon for augmentative
      communication, 230
Social skills
   communicative competence in,
      50–51
   in emotionally handicapped, 130
   lexical items in augmentative
      communication fostering, 226

Social skills—*continued*
  techniques for teaching, 52
Speak and spell toys, 238
Specificity, language facilitation by,
    108
Speech awareness increase,
    spontaneous language
    decreased by, 154–157
Speech synthesizer, of
    microcomputers, 237–238
Spontaneous imitation, as language
    facilitation strategy, 113
Spontaneous language, 145–146
  atmosphere of delight in, 160–161
  blocking, 155
  communicative interplay in,
    155–157
  context and, 158–159
  environmental demands and,
    154–155
  fitting the person, 157–158
  increase in speech awareness
    decreasing, 154–157
  laughter and, 154, 161
  pumping and, 154–155, 156–157,
    161
  unconscious generation of,
    146–153
Stimulus pictures, in aphasia
    treatment, 186–187
Stimulus presentation, manner of for
    emotionally handicapped, 143
Stimulus-response intervention
    technique, 2–3
  packaged programs, 5–7
  see also Developmental approach
Strategies of learning, 46, 61
  attention, 68–69
  discrimination, 70
  for language curriculum, 67–71
  for language development, 29
  matching, 69
  relationship between children's
    and instructor's, 70–71
  see also Imitation
Stress, language performance and,
    154
Structured observation, as language
    assessment procedure, 75, 76
Structured play treatment session, 8
Subject, in a three-constituent
    utterance, 19

Support systems, need for, 52–53
Symbolic play, 82, 84
Symbol sets
  Amerind, 226
  Blissymbolics, 218–219, 222, 226
  selection procedures, 206
  see also Augmentative
    communication
Syntax
  assessment, 46–47, 86
  development of, 80–81
  in emotionally handicapped,
    127–128
  language intervention and, 51

Tape recorder, competing auditory
    messages of the classroom
    simulated by, 50
Task analysis, data based language
    programs and, 15–16
Task repetition, for emotionally
    handicapped children, 137
Test of Basic Concepts, 49
Tests and testing
  Boston Diagnostic Aphasia Exam,
    176
  in classroom, 49
  in clinic, 49
  Communication Activities of
    Daily Living, 177
  of comprehension and production,
    46–53
  criterion referenced, 64–67
  error in design and structure of,
    64
  for fluent aphasics, 176–177
  formal, 73, 76
  informal, 73
  interactive model and, 81–86
  of language improvement, 73–76
  microcomputers for, 238–241, 245
  norm referenced, 64
  picture pointing tasks for, 47
  Porch Index of Communicative
    Ability, 176
  readiness, 48
  Receptive Expressive Emergent
    Language Scale, 82
  recognition for, 47
  Sequenced Inventory of
    Communication
    Development, 82

Test of Basic Concepts, 49
Uzgiris-Hunt Scales of
    Psychological Development,
    82
Three-word utterance level,
    treatment approach for child
    with, 92–93
Time, coding, 110
Tokens, as reinforcement, 6
Tool use, 82, 84
Topic sharing, 105
Transitive verbs, 32–33
Turns, withholding, 111
Tutors, 52–53
Two-word stage
    assessment during, 83, 85–86, 87
    treatment approach for child at,
    90–91

Uncontractible auxiliary,
    development of, 3, 6–7
Uncontractible copula, development
    of, 3–4
Unknowing compensator, fluent
    aphasic as, 174–176
Use, 80
    in Bloom-Lahey model, 125–126
    contextual components affecting,
    99–100
    model, see Communicative
    context
    in emotionally handicapped child,
    133, 134
    disorders, 128–129
Uzgiris-Hunt Scales of
    Psychological Development,
    82

Verbs
    in aphasia treatment, 186
    catenatives, 112, 114–115
    causative, 32–33
    infinitives, 111

intransitive, 32–33
past tense, 3–4
"s" in, 34–35
third person singular, 3–4
transitive, 32–33
see also Auxiliaries; Progressive
    endings
Vertical developmental approach, to
    language training, 3–4
Vignettes, for social awareness, 52
Visual imagery, treatment of aphasia
    with, 184
Visual-spatial-holistic deblocker,
    191, 193, 195–196, 198, 199,
    200, 201, 202
Vocabulary building,
    microcomputers for, 243–244
Vocabulary comprehension, 71
Vocal imitation, 82, 84
Votrax, of microcomputers, 237–238

Wernicke's aphasia, 166, 189, 190,
    192–193
    deblocking, 197–202
Wernicke's aprosodia, 189
Wh-questions, 112, 114–115
Wilson Initial Syntax Program
    (WISP), 238
WISP, see Wilson Initial Syntax
    Program
Word pool, for augmentative
    communication, 214–217
Word retrieval problem, in
    emotionally handicapped
    children, 127
Working alliance, with emotionally
    handicapped child, 123–125,
    134–135

Young children, assessment and
    treatment of language delay
    in, see Interactive model